NEW DRUGS, CONCEPTS AND RESULTS IN CANCER CHEMOTHERAPY

Cancer Treatment and Rcscarch

WILLIAM L MCGUIRE, *series editor*

Livingston, RB (ed): Lung Cancer 1. 1981. ISBN 90-247-2394-9.
Humphrey GB, Dehner LP, Grindey GB, Acton RT (eds): Pediatric Oncology 1. ISBN 90-274-2408-2.
DeCosse JJ, Sherlock P (eds): Gastrointestinal Cancer 1. 1981. ISBN 90-247-2461-9.
Bennett JM (ed): Lymphomas 1, including Hodgkin's Disease. 1981. ISBN 90-247-2479-1.
Bloomfield CD (ed): Adult Leukemias 1. 1982. ISBN 90-247-2478-3.
Paulson DF (ed): Genitourinary Cancer 1. 1982. ISBN 90-247-2480-5.
Muggia FM (ed): Cancer Chemotherapy 1. 1983. ISBN 90-247-2713-8.
Humphrey GB, Grindey GB (eds): Pancreatic Tumors in Children. 1982. ISBN 90-247-2702-2.
Costanzi JJ (ed): Malignant Melanoma 1. 1983. ISBN 90-247-2706-5.
Griffiths CT, Fuller AF (eds): Gynecologic Oncology. 1983. ISBN 0-89838-555-5.
Greco AF (ed): Biology and Management of Lung Cancer. 1983. ISBN 0-89838-554-7.
Walker M.D. (ed): Oncology of the Nervous System. 1983. ISBN 0-89839-567-9.
Higby D.J. (ed): Supportive Care in Cancer Therapy. 1983. ISBN 0-89838-569-5.
Herberman R.B. (ed): Basic and Clinical Tumor Immunology. 1983. ISBN 0-89838-579-2.
Baker LH (ed): Soft Tissue Sarcomas. 1983. ISBN 0-89838-584-9.
Bennett JM (ed): Controversies in the Management of Lymphomas. 1983. ISBN 0-89838-586-5.
Humphrey GB, Grindey GB (eds): Adrenal and Endocrine Tumors in Children. 1983. ISBN 0-89838-590-3.
DeCosse JJ, Sherlock P. (eds): Clinical Management of Gastrointestinal Cancer. 1984. ISBN 0-89838-601-2.
Catalona WJ, Ratliff TL (eds): Urologic Oncology. 1984. ISBN 0-89838-628-4.
Santen RJ, Manni A (eds): Diagnosis and Management of Endocrine-Related Tumors. 1984. ISBN 0-89838-636-5.
Costanzi JJ (ed): Clinical Management of Malignant Melanoma. 1984. ISBN 0-89838-656-X.
Wolf GT (ed): Head and Neck Oncology. 1984. ISBN 0-89838-657-8.
Alberts DS, Surwit EA (eds): Ovarian Cancer. 1985. ISBN 0-89838-676-4.
Muggia FM (ed): Experimental and Clinical Progress in Cancer Chemotherapy. 1985. ISBN 0-89838-679-9.
Higby DJ (ed): Issues in Supportive Care of Cancer Patients. 1986. ISBN 0-89838-816-3.
Surwit EA, Alberts DS (eds): Cervix Cancer. 1987. ISBN 0-89838-822-8.
Jacobs C (ed): Cancers of the Head and Neck. 1987. ISBN 0-89838-825-2.
MacDonald JS (ed): Gastrointestinal Oncology. 1987. ISBN 0-89838-829-5.
Ratliff TL, Catalona WJ (eds): Genitourinary Cancer. 1987. ISBN 0-89838-830-9.
Nathanson L (ed): Basic and Clinical Aspects of Malignant Melanoma. 1987. ISBN 0-89838-856-2.
Muggia FM (ed): Concepts, Clinical Developments, and Therapeutic Advances in Cancer Chemotherapy. 1987. ISBN 0-89838-897-5.
Frankel AE (ed): Immunotoxins. 1988. ISBN 0-89838-984-4.
Bennett JM, Foon KA (eds): Immunologic Approaches to the Classification and Management of Lymphomas and Leukemias. 1988. ISBN 0-89838-355-2.
Osborne CK (ed): Endocrine Therapies in Breast and Prostate Cancer. 1988. ISBN 0-89838-365-X.
Lippman ME, Dickson R (eds): Breast Cancer: Cellular and Molecular Biology. 1988. ISBN 0-89838-368-4.
Kamps WA, Humphrey GB, Poppema S (eds): Hodgkin's Disease in Children: Controversies and Current Practice. 1988. ISBN 0-89838-372-2.
Muggia FM (ed): Cancer Chemotherapy: Concepts, Clinical Investigations and Therapeutic Advances. 1988. ISBN 0-89838-381-1.
Nathanson L (ed): Malignant Melanoma: Biology, Diagnosis, and Therapy. 1988. ISBN 0-89838-384-6.
Pinedo HM, Verweij J (eds): Treatment of Soft Tissue Sarcomas. 1989. ISBN 0-89838-391-9.
Hansen HH (ed): Basic and Clinical Concepts of Lung Cancer. 1989. ISBN 0-7923-0153-6.
Lepor H., Ratliff TL (eds): Urologic Oncology. 1989. ISBN 0-7923-0161-7.
Benz C., Liu E. (eds): Oncogenes. 1989. ISBN 0-7923-0237-0.
Ozols RF (ed): Drug Resistance in Cancer Therapy. 1989. ISBN 0-7923-0244-3.
Surwit EA, Alberts DS (eds): Endometrial Cancer. 1989. ISBN 0-7923-0286-9.
Champlin R (ed): Bone Marrow Transplantation. 1990. ISBN 0-7923-0612-0.
Goldenberg D. (ed): Cancer Imaging with Radiolabeled Antibodies. 1990. ISBN 0-7923-0631-7.
Jacobs C. (ed): Carcinomas of the Head and Neck. 1990. ISBN 0-7923-0668-6.
Lippman M.E., Dickson R. (eds): Regulatory Mechanisms in Breast Cancer: Advances in Cellular and Molecular Biology of Breast Cancer. 1990. ISBN 0-7923-0868-9.
Nathanson, L. (ed): Maligant Melanoma: Genetics, Growth Factors, Metastases, and Antigens. 1991. ISBN 0-7923-0895-6.
Sugarbaker, PH (ed): Management of Gastric Cancer. 1991. ISBN 0-7923-1102-7.
Pinedo HM, Verweij J, Suit, HD, (eds): Soft Tissue Sarcomas: New Developments in the Multidisciplinary Approach to Treatment. ISBN 0-7923-1139-6.
Ozols, RF, (ed): Molecular and Clinical Advances in Anticancer Drug Resistance. 1991. ISBN 0-7923-1212-0.
Muggia, FM (ed): New Drugs, Concepts and Results in Cancer Chemotherapy 1991. ISBN

New Drugs, Concepts and Results in Cancer Chemotherapy

Edited by

F.M. MUGGIA
University of Southern California Cancer Center

1991 **KLUWER ACADEMIC PUBLISHERS**
BOSTON / DORDRECHT / LONDON

Distributors
for North America: Kluwer Academic Publishers, 101 Philip Drive, Assinippi Park, Norwell, Massachusetts 02061 USA

for all other countries: Kluwer Academic Publishers Group, Distribution Centre, Post Office Box 322, 3300 AH Dordrecht, THE NETHERLANDS

Cancer Treatment and Reseach is indexed in the National Library of Medicine MEDLARS system.

Library of Congress Cataloging-in-Publication Data

New drugs, concepts, and results in cancer chemotherapy/edited by F.M. Muggia.
p. cm.—(Cancer treatment and research; v. 58)
Includes bibliographical references and index.
ISBN 0-7923-1253-8
1. Antineoplastic agents. 2. Cancer—Chemotherapy. I. Muggia, Franco M. II. Series.
[DNLM: 1. Antineoplastic Agents—pharmacology. 2. Antineoplastic Agents—therapeutic use. 3. Neoplasms—drug therapy. W1 CA693 v. 58/QV 269 N5323]
RC271.C5N465 1991
616.99′4061—dc20
DNLM/DLC
for Library of Congress 91-7085
CIP

Cancer Treatment and Research is indexed in the National Library of Medicine *MEDLARS* System.

PRINTED IN THE UNITED STATES OF AMERICA.

Printed on acid-free paper.

Table of Contents

List of Contributors

PEGGY ALDERTON, M.D., The Royal Melbourne Hospital, University of Melbourne, Parkville, Victoria 3050, Australia

RODRIGO ARRIAGADA, 39, rue Camille Desmoulins, Institut Gustave-Roussy, 94805 Villejuif, France

AVI I. EINZIG, M.D., Albert Einstein College of Medicine, 111 East 210th St., Bronx, NY 10467

RAKESH GOEL, M.D., Department of Medicine, T-012, University of California, San Diego Cancer Center, La Jolla, CA 92093

MICHAEL D. GREEN, M.D., The Royal Melbourne Hospital, University of Melbourne, Parkville, Victoria 3050, Australia

JANET GROSS, M.D., The Royal Melbourne Hospital, University of Melbourne, Parkville, Victoria 3050, Australia

STEVEN M. GRUNBERG, M.D., Division of Medical Oncology, University of Southern California, Comprehensive Cancer Center, 1441 Eastlake Avenue, Los Angeles, CA 90033

JOHN S. HOLCENBERG, M.D., Vice President and Director Clinical Affairs, Immunex Research and Development Corp., 51 University Street, Seattle, WA 98101

STEPHEN B. HOWELL, M.D., Division of Hematology/Oncology, Department of Medicine, T-012, University of California, San Diego Cancer Center, La Jolla, CA 92093

FRANK P. LaCRETA, Fox Chase Cancer Center, 7701 Burholme Avenue, Philadelphia, PA 19111

THIERRY LE CHEVALIER, M.D., 39, rue Camille Desmoulins, Institut Gustave-Roussy, 94805 Villejuif, France

PATRICK J. LOEHRER, Indiana University, School of Medicine, 926 W. Michigan, Indianapolis, IN 46223

RICHARD G. MORAN, Ph.D., Depts. of Biochemistry, Pediatrics, and Pharmacy and Norris Cancer Center, University of Southern California, Los Angeles, CA 90033

FRANCO M. MUGGIA, M.D., Kenneth Norris Jr. Comprehensive Cancer Center, 1441 Eastlake Avenue, Los Angeles, CA 90033

NIKHIL C. MUNSHI, Indiana University, School of Medicine, 926 W. Michigan, Indianapolis, IN 46223

PETER J. O'DWYER, Fox Chase Cancer Center, 7701 Burholme Avenue, Philadelphia, PA 19111

EDWARD L. SCHWARTZ, M.D., Albert Einstein College of Medicine, 111 East 210th Street, Bronx, NY 10467

MORDECHAI M. SOBOL, M.D., The Royal Melbourne Hospital, University of Melbourne, Parkville, Victoria 3050, Australia

JAMES L. SPEYER, M.D., Division of Oncology, New York University Medical Center, New York, NY 10016

MAURICE TUBIANA, 39, rue Camille Desmoulins, institut Gustave-Roussy, 94805 Villejuif, France

PETER H. WIERNIK, M.D., Department of Oncology, Montefiore Medical Center, Albert Einstein College of Medicine, 111 East 210th Street, Bronx, NY 10467

STEPHEN D. WILLIAMS, M.D., Indiana University, School of Medicine, 926 W. Michigan, Indianapolis, IN 46223

HENRY P. WU, Departments of Pediatrics and Biochemistry, University of Southern California, Childrens Hospital Los Angeles, Los Angeles, CA 90054

Cancer Treatment and Research

Foreword to the Series

Where do you begin to look for a recent, authoritative article on the diagnosis or management of a particular malignancy? The few general oncology textbooks are generally out of date. Single papers in specialized journals are informative but seldom comprehensive; these are more often preliminary reports on a very limited number of patients. Certain general journals frequently publish good in-depth reviews of cancer topics, and published symposium lectures are often the best overviews available. Unfortunately, these reviews and supplements appear sporadically, and the reader can never be sure when a topic of special interest will be covered.

Cancer Treatment and Research is a series of authoritative volumes that aim to meet this need. It is an attempt to establish a critical mass of oncology literature covering virtually all oncology topics, revised frequently to keep the coverage up to date, and easily available on a single library shelf or by a single personal subscription.

We have approached the problem in the following fashion: first, by dividing the oncology literature into specific subdivisions, such as lung cancer, genitourinary cancer, pediatric oncology, etc.; and second, by asking eminent authorities in each of these areas to edit a volume on the specific topic on an annual or biannual basis. Each topic and tumor type is covered in a volume appearing frequently and predictably, discussing current diagnosis, staging, markers, all forms of treatment modalities, basic biology, and more.

In *Cancer Treatment and Research*, we have an outstanding group of editors, each having made a major commitment to bring to this new series the very best literature in his or her field. Kluwer Academic Publishers has made an equally major commitment to the rapid publication of high-quality books and to worldwide distribution.

Where can you go to find quickly a recent authoritative article on any major oncology problem? We hope that *Cancer Treatment and Research* provides an answer.

WILLIAM L. MCGUIRE
Series Editor

Preface

The decade of the 1990s will see an increasing emphasis on the modulation of chemotherapeutic drug selectivity and in the 'lock and key' approach to new targets to control malignant proliferation. The contents of this volume appropriately reflect these scientific undercurrents.

An emerging powerful tool of molecular pharmacology is described by Holcenberg and Wu. Manipulation of genetic expression by modification of messenger RNA is now within our reach, and the basic concepts are succinctly reviewed as a primer on future biochemical engineering of new anticancer molecules. Another concept that appears to be worthy of further study in both experimental and clinical chemotherapy concerns observations on the modulation of activity by the nucleoside transport inhibitor, dipyridamole. How potentiation of several anticancer drugs occurs has practical, as well as theoretical, ramifications, discussed by Goel and Howell. Finally, O'Dwyer and La Creta present a fresh look at sensitization of chemotherapy by the hypoxic radiosensitizer, SR-2731.

Moran describes the biochemistry of the folate analog 5, 10 dideazatetrahydrofolate (DDATHF), which has been the recent subject of clinical Phase I study by our group. This drug emerges as one of the most potent antimetabolites ever introduced. The other two drugs discussed are modifiers that have achieved a clinical spotlight because of their capability to reverse troublesome toxicities of commonly used drugs. Green and colleagues discuss doxorubicin—the cardioprotector ICRF-187, while Munshi and colleagues provide practical tips on the use of the uroprotector mesna with the escalating doses of oxazaphosphorines being given clinically. The availability of mesna is providing new therapeutic opportunities for both cyclophosphamide and ifosfamide, which will be further strengthened by colony stimulating factors and autologous bone marrow or peripheral stem cell reconstitution.

Disease targets covered include the often neglected meningiomas, and small-cell lung cancer. The study of hormone receptors in meningioma has opened the way for new therapeutic approaches—truly an example of trying to find the right key to control the growth of this tumor, as demonstrated by Grunberg's clinical studies. Lastly, the conventional approaches of radiation and chemotherapy, given intensively in interdigitating schedules, are associated with convincingly better results. This malignancy has been a target of therapeutic study in the past three decades after chemosensitivity and radiosensitivity were discovered. The trials at Gustave-Roussy described by LeChevalier illustrate the success that may be achieved.

The contents of this volume are an appropriate opening for this new decade. Undoubtedly, we enter an era of refinement of current treatment as well as of discovery and application of powerful new tools.

NEW DRUGS, CONCEPTS AND RESULTS IN CANCER CHEMOTHERAPY

1. Pharmacologic control of specific gene expression

John S. Holcenberg and Henry P. Wu

Introduction

Cancer cells proliferate, invade surrounding tissues, and metastasize because they have escaped the normal mechanisms that control these processes [1, 2]. Many of the genes that regulate these processes have now been isolated and characterized. Pharmacologic control of the expression of these genes would provide exciting new approaches to cancer chemotherapy.

A major advance in the understanding of carcinogenesis was the discovery that certain retroviruses contain *oncogenes*, genes that can induce cancers after infection of normal cells. Cellular homologs of these viral oncogenes, called *protooncogenes*, were discovered in normal cells through experiments with viral infection and transfection of DNA fragments. Protooncogenes encode growth factors, growth factor receptors, signal transducers of growth factors, and nuclear factors that control DNA replication or gene expression. Protooncogenes induce cancers when their products are mutated, expressed in excess amount, or expressed at abnormal times in the cell cycle or in ontogeny [3–5]. In addition to known human protooncogenes, some cancer cells escape normal growth control by increased production of growth factors or growth factor receptors, or by loss of response to negative regulatory factors [6]. Many of these protooncogenes and growth factors have now been cloned and characterized.

Recently, recessive genes have been discovered that can suppress tumor formation [7, 8]. Loss or inactivation of both alleles of these *antioncogenes* or *suppressor* genes is a causal factor in tumorigenesis of retinoblastoma, Wilms' tumor, and osteogenic sarcomas in children, and may contribute to tumor formation in adult tumors. The product of the retinoblastoma suppressor gene has recently been shown to interact with transforming proteins of DNA tumor viruses [9]. Cancers may arise by loss of the suppressor effects of the retinoblastoma gene when it binds with the viral protein. Thus, cancers may result from an imbalance between factors that promote growth and factors that inhibit growth and lead to differentiation.

One of the major processes in the spread and metastasis of cancers is their invasion of basement membranes and connective tissues. Certain cells

Franco M. Muggia (ed.), NEW DRUGS, CONCEPTS AND RESULTS IN CANCER CHEMOTHERAPY.

Kluwer Academic Publishers, Boston. *ISBN 0-7923-1253-8*

produce and secrete plasminogen activators, collagenases, and other proteolytic enzymes that catalyze the degradation of surrounding tissues. Normally, this degradation of supporting tissue is controlled by the secretion of inhibitors of these enzymes by the same cells or other cells in the tissue. Tumor cell invasion may be due to alterations in the balance of these factors [10].

The growth and invasion of cancer cells could be arrested by agents that turn on or off specific genes that control these processes. Agents under investigation include synthetic polymers and oligonucleotides that bind to DNA, antisense oligonucleotides that bind to messenger RNA, and double-stranded oligonucleotides that compete for nuclear binding factors. Such therapies may be able to decrease the expression of oncogenes, tumor growth factors, growth factor receptors, or enzymes that facilitate the invasion of cancer cells. Alternatively, this therapy might be able to increase the expression of tumor suppressor genes or other factors that inhibit growth, induce differentiation, or inhibit tumor invasion.

This chapter will review the current status of these efforts to construct agents that interact with specific sites on DNA, RNA, and nuclear regulatory proteins. In each case the potential therapy will be judged for a) its specificity of binding to the target, b) its stability in plasma and cells, and c) its ability to cross cellular membranes. These approaches are not yet ready for clinical testing, but they may be part of cancer treatment in the next decade.

DNA-binding polymers and oligonucleotides

The intercalating anticancer drugs, doxorubicin, actinomycin D, m-AMSA, and mitoxantrone, have some selectivity for guanine/cytosine (G-C)-rich regions of double-stranded DNA, while bleomycin binds preferentially to adenine-thymidine (A-T)-rich regions [11]. Greater specificity is seen with the polymeric natural products, netropsin and distamycin, which bind to A-T-rich regions in the minor groove of DNA. Figure 1 shows the structure of distamycin; the curved backbone of this polymer fits the minor groove of the DNA helix. The selectivity is due to tight van der Waals contact between the pyrrole residues of these polymers and the nucleotide bases that allows binding between A-T base pairs but prevents binding to the bulkier G-C base pairs [12]. Goodsell and Dickerson [13] have shown that substitution of the residues in these polymers with imidazole groups leads to preferential binding to G-C-rich regions due to hydrogen bonding to guanine residues. By synthesizing a specific sequence of residues, it should be possible to make a drug with specificity for a selected order of G-C and A-T base pairs in double-stranded DNA. Residues that would bind preferentially to A-T base pairs include pyrrole and benzyl residues; imidazole, furan, or pyrimidine groups would hydrogen bond and bind preferentially to G-C base pairs. These sequence-reading synthetic polymers, called *isolexins*, would have

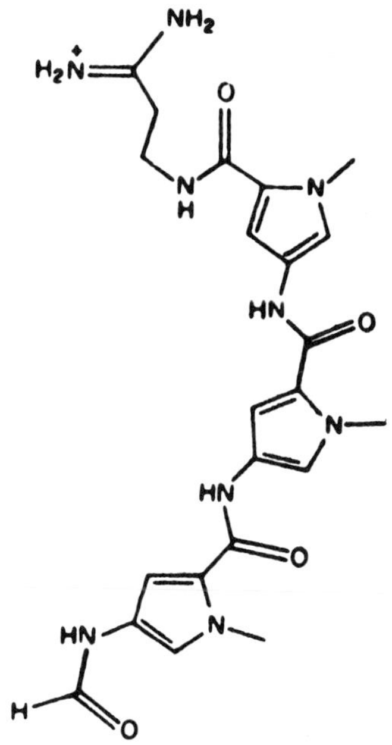

Figure 1. Structure of distamycin.

only *half* specificity, since the polymer cannot discriminate between an A-T vs. T-A or a G-C vs. a C-G base pair in the DNA duplex.

Recent studies with three minor groove binders, distamycin A, bisbenzimide (Hoechst 33258), and 4′,6-diamidino-2-phenylindole, indicate that they alter topoisomerase I and II activity [14, 15]. Thus, they may be useful in combination therapy with drugs that interact with topoisomerases.

Dervan and coworkers [16] have expanded the therapeutic possibilities of these polymers by covalently linking functional groups like EDTA-Fe(II) and thereby introducing DNA cleavage at specific sites. Krowiski et al. [17] have shown increased specificity of alkylating agents by covalently binding them to these polymers. Little is known about the transport of these polymers across cell membranes or their pharmacology in whole animals. Upjohn Company has isolated analogues of the antibiotic CC-1065 that covalently bind in the minor groove. These compounds are not cross-resistant to distamycin, netropsin, or other known DNA binding anticancer drugs [18].

An alternative to DNA-binding polymers is the use of oligonucleotides, which hydrogen bond to complimentary sequences of DNA or RNA with high specificity. It has been estimated that an oligonucleotide of 17 bases will hybridize with only one sequence in human DNA. Thus, relatively short oligonucleotides can bind specific regions of single-stranded DNA or RNA.

Addition of functional groups to these oligonucleotides can cause cleavage or irreversible binding to a specific target sequence.

The reaction rates of nitrogen mustard drugs with guanine-N7 groups of DNA differ depending on the electrostatic potential of their nearest neighbor nucleotides in a DNA sequence [19]. Further specificity towards single-stranded DNA has been achieved by linking nitrogen mustard, platinum, or EDTA-Fe(II) groups to short oligonucleotides that are complementary to the DNA [20–23].

There probably are very few regions of DNA with sufficient single-stranded character for a short single-stranded oligonucleotide to compete for binding with the opposite strand of the DNA. Surprisingly, oligonucleotides have been shown to interact with double-stranded DNA. Moser and Dervan [23] have demonstrated that an EDTA-Fe(II) homopyrimidine oligonucleotide can form a triple helix with a double-stranded homopurine-homopyrimidine DNA sequence in vitro and cause cleavage at specific sites. The third strand binds by Hoogsteen base pairing in the major groove of the DNA helix [24]. Similar results have been reported with oligonucleotides linked to a copper-phenanthroline complex [25]. Helene and coworkers [26] have used oligonucleotides linked to intercalating acridine dyes as sequence-specific probes. The intercalating agent stabilizes the complex when it is separated from the oligonucleotide by a five- or six-carbon methylene group spacer. Recently, this group has shown sequence-specific cleavage when a homopyrimidine oligonucleotide linked to ellipticine is photoactivated [27]. These compounds will have much greater specificity than the minor groove binding polymers. In contrast, they will be susceptible to degradation by nucleases and have limited transport across cellular membranes due to the negative charge on the phosphate groups. Chemical modifications that can stabilize oligonucleotides and increase their transport are discussed in the next section.

Antisense RNA-binding oligonucleotides

Antisense oligonucleotides are RNA or DNA sequences that are complementary to messenger RNA. Their binding to particular mRNA sequences blocks translation into protein. Antisense RNA (also called *micRNA* for mRNA interfering complementary RNA) is produced naturally in certain bacteria in response to changes in growth conditions [28]. In 1978, Zamecnik and Stephensen [29] demonstrated that a 13-mer oligonucleotide complementary to the terminal repeat of Rous sarcoma virus 35S RNA could inhibit transformation, replication, and translation of this virus in chicken embryo fibroblasts. This work stimulated great interest in oligonucleotides as therapeutic agents to block expression of specific genes, since it demonstrated that these charged molecules can be taken up by cells and have biologic effects. Comprehensive reviews of antisense oligonucleotides have been published [30–32], so we will discuss only the major experiments that address their mechanisms of action, efficacy, specificity, stability, transport across cell membranes, and whole-animal experiments.

Early experiments used either microinjection or transfection to introduce antisense RNA or DNA into cells. Melton [33] injected frog oocytes with purified mRNAs that encode β-globin and various antisense portions for this gene. Synthesis of β-globin protein was maximally blocked if the eggs were first injected with the antisense RNA and if the antisense RNA included the 5′ region of the gene. The antisense RNA was unstable if it did not contain an mRNA cap structure. This method could inhibit specific genes in early embryos, since these eggs do not synthesize new RNA. Since later embryos or mature cells might synthesize RNA that would dilute out the effect of antisense RNA, a single injection would not be effective. Some more mature cells also contain an enzyme that unwinds RNA-RNA duplexes and decreases the inhibition by the antisense RNA [34]. To overcome these problems, Izant and Weintraub [35] microinjected plasmids with strong promoters that could produce a continuous supply of a specific antisense RNA. Plasmids containing both sense and antisense orientations of herpes simplex thymidine kinase (TK) were injected into mouse L cells lacking this enzyme. Expression of TK was significantly decreased when the cells were injected with a 10 to 100-fold excess of antisense DNA to sense DNA. The inhibition was sequence specific and was seen with antisense constructs as small as 52 base pairs and with fragments complementary to either the protein coding or the 5′ untranslated regions. Similar effects were seen when the plasmids were introduced into the cells by calcium phosphate transfection or when other promoters and reporter genes were used [36].

Kim and Wold showed that antisense TK could also inhibit expression of endogenous TK in mouse L cells [37]. These cells were stably transfected with a plasmid that contained both antisense TK and sense dihydrofolate reductase. Cells expressing high levels of dihydrofolate reductase would be resistant to the antifolate methotrexate. Since both genes are on the same plasmid, cells selected for methotrexate resistance should express high levels of antisense TK. Analysis of many clones of these transfected L cells showed that the ratio of antisense to sense RNA had to be at least 100:1 to reduce TK expression by 80–90%. RNA-RNA duplexes were found in the nucleus, suggesting that the inhibition was due to prevention of RNA processing or translocation of the pre-mRNA to the cytoplasm. Despite the 10-fold reduction in TK activity, these cells still had enough residual enzyme activity to be sensitive to bromodeoxyuridine, a drug that requires TK for activity. Similar results were obtained when human HL-60 cells expressing high levels of antisense *c-myc* were selected with HAT media and mycophenolic acid [38]. A 10 to 25-fold excess of antisense to sense DNA and RNA was needed to decrease expression of *c-myc* protein and the growth rate of these cells.

In another example, antisense RNA was shown to alter the phenotype of developing Drosophila embryos [39]. The embryos were injected with sense and antisense RNA of the Kruppel gene, a gene needed for segmentation. The percentage of embryos with abnormal development increased with the amount of antisense RNA injected. Thus, expression of antisense transcripts of single genes can block a complex program of development.

Antisense RNAs have also been designed to prevent infections. When bacteria were stably transfected with plasmids containing antisense constructs of genes required for replication of a phage, they were resistant to infection by this phage [40]. Similarly, tissue culture cells were made resistant to retroviral infection when they were transformed by a retrovirus containing an antisense construct to a gene in the infecting virus [41]. In the future this approach may be used to transfect bone marrow and lymphoid progenitor cells in vitro. Injection of the transfected cells into the host would confer an intracellular immunity to a specific virus in this population.

These experiments using microinjection or transfection have suggested that several mechanisms may be involved in the inhibition of gene expression when antisense oligonucleotides hybridize to RNA. The sequence specificity and preference for the 5′ regions of the RNA suggest that the oligonucleotide-RNA duplex blocks or arrests translation [42, 43]. Other experiments indicate that the duplexes trap the mRNA in the nucleus [37] or they are substrates for RNAase H, an enzyme that cleaves DNA-RNA duplexes [44, 45].

Although these methods have been useful for studying antisense, microinjection, plasmid transfection, and retroviral infection have limited applications as techniques to introduce antisense oligonucleotides into cells. Microinjected RNA has a short duration of action in mature cells. Microinjected plasmids must be integrated into the host's genome for stable expression. This integration is random and could lead to altered expression of critical genes in the host. Plasmid transfection requires harsh conditions, such as $CaCl_2$, DEAE-dextran, lipid encapsulation, or electroporation to introduce the large circular DNA into the cells. Furthermore, techniques are not available to transfect plasmids into selective cells in a whole animal. Infection with retroviruses containing the antisense construct can effectively introduce DNA into cells, but it is currently impossible to control the extent of the infection in a whole organism and the DNA is randomly inserted into the genome.

An alternative method is to expose cells to short linear antisense oligonucleotides that can be taken up by cells. This approach has be used to block the expression of specific genes. For example, exposure of human T cells to 30 μM concentrations of a 15-mer containing antisense *c-myc* prevented entry of the cells into S phase after stimulation with PHA [46]. Similarly, DNA synthesis and mitosis were suppressed by incubation of cells with 18-mer antisense oligonucleotides to PCNA, a cofactor of DNA polymerases [47]. These experiments were carried out in media containing heat-inactivated serum that lacks the usual nucleases found in serum. More stable oligonucleotide derivatives may be needed for activity in animals.

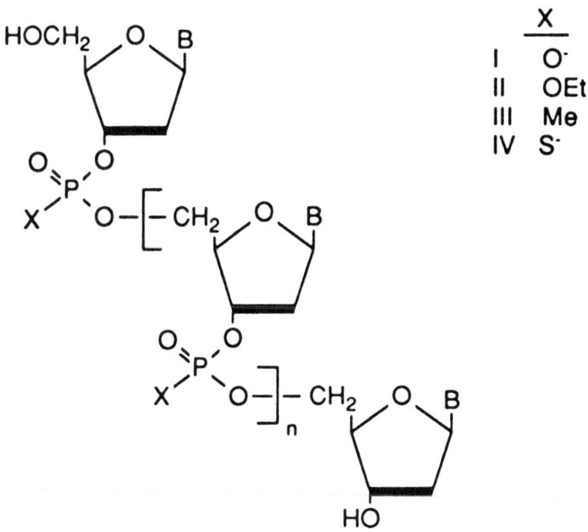

Figure 2. Structure of normal and modified oligonucleotides. B represents nucleic acid bases. I is the normal phosphate linkage, II is a ethyl-phosphotriester, III is a methylphosphonate, and IV is a phosphorothioate. (Reproduced from Abramova et al. [22], with permission.)

Table 1. Characteristics of oligonucleotide derivatives

Name	*X*	*Nuclease*	*Stereoisomers*	*Hydrophobicity*	*Aqueous solubility*
Normal, phosphodiester	O	Sensitive	No		High
Ethyl phosphotriester	OCH_2CH_3	Resistant[a]	Yes	Increased	Low
Methyl phosphonate	CH_3	Resistant	Yes	Increased	Low
Phosphorothioate	S-	Resistant	Yes		High

* Deethylated in cells, then degraded.

The major derivatives that have been investigated are alkyl-phosphotriesters, methylphosphonates, phosphorothioates, α-oligonucleotides, and normal phosphodiesters linked to polymers or intercalators. Figure 2 shows the general structure of the first three derivatives. Table 1 shows some of their properties. The first three derivatives differ from normal phosphodiester-linked oligonucleotides by alternations in one of the substituents on the phosphorus. Alkyl phosphotriesters and methylphosphonates do not carry the normal negative charge on the phosphorus, so they have increased lipid solubility, possibly increased permeability into cells, and tighter binding to polynucleotide targets at low salt concentrations. At physiologic salt concentrations this binding advantage for the non-ionic analogues should be minimal [32]. All these derivatives are more resistant to nucleases, except the alkyl phosphotriesters, which are hydrolyzed to phosphodiesters in cells and then degraded.

Another class of oligonucleotides has α linkages between the bases and the sugar, rather than the natural β linkage. These α-oligonucleotides are stable to nuclease digestion and form parallel, rather than antiparallel, duplexes with B-DNA. These compounds can now be synthesized on authomated machines, so they may be tested more extensively as antisense agents. The α-oligonucleotides can be made with phosphorothioate linkages, which would add further resistance to degradation in cells [32].

The substitutions on the phosphorus are asymmetrical. Therefore, chemical syntheses of these derivatives lead to random orientations of stereoisomers. For an oligomer of length n there will be $2^{(n-1)}$ stereoisomers. When these oligonucleotide derivatives form double-stranded structures with their target, the substituent can be oriented either towards or away from the helix. The inward orientation may destabilize the helix due to steric hindrance. This causes a decrease in melting temperature (T_m) of the duplex of 4–12° for 11 to 14-oligomer analogues compared to the normal phosphodiesters of the same sequence [32]. This effect may lower the T_m to less than 37° for short oligonucleotides with a high percentage of A-T nucleotides and lead to decreased equilibrium binding to targets in cells under physiological conditions.

The synthesis and characterization of oligonucleotide derivatives were pioneered by Miller and Ts'o [48, 49]. They showed that a methylphosphonate deoxythymidine octamer was taken up by Syrian fibroblasts and that less than 30% was degraded in 18 hours. In contrast, ethyl-phosphotriesters were converted to the phosphodiesters and degraded. Short methylphosphonate oligonucleotides were shown to specifically inhibit translation of rabbit α and β globin genes in cell-free and whole-cell models. Miller and coworkers [50] designed methylphosphonate oligonucleotides that bind to the splice junctions of viral pre-RNA. Viral titers were decreased 90% when HSV I-infected cells were incubated with 75 μM or more of an 8-mer complementary to an acceptor splice junction of HSV type I mRNAs 4 and 5. This antisense methylphosphonate was also effective when applied as a cream to an HSV lesion on the ear. Recently, a 30 μM concentration of a 15-mer methylphosphonate containing the initiation codon of the multiple drug resistance gene, *MDR1*, was shown to inhibit production of this protein and to partially reverse daunomycin resistance in K562 erythroleukemia cells [53]. In order to decrease the effective concentrations of the antisense oligonucleotides, Miller and coworkers [51, 52] have attached trimethylpsoralen to methylphosphonate. Exposure of the cells to light photoactivated the psoralen derivative, cross-linked the oligonucleotide to the target, and produced inhibition of specific protein synthesis at 5 μM.

Initially the methylphosphonates were synthesized stepwise on insoluble polystyrene supports using protected 5′-dimethoxytrityl-deoxyribonucleoside

3′-methylphosphonic imidazolides as synthetic intermediates. Now methods are available to produce them in larger amounts on a DNA synthesizer [32, 53]. One disadvantage of the methylphosphonates is their poor water solubility; this property precludes use of very long derivatives of this type. Duplexes of methylphosphonate oligonucleotides and RNA are not substrates for RNAase H [32].

Phosphorothioate derivatives have several advantages over other derivatives as antisense agents. They can be synthesized easily by automated machines. Currently, their nucleotide sequence is assembled from hydrogen-phosphonate monomers and then converted to the phosphorothioates in a single-step reaction [54]. Phosphorothioates are negatively charged, like phosphodiesters, but they are highly resistant to nuclease degradation. Like phosphodiesters, duplexes of phosphorothioates and RNA are substrates for RNAase H [32]. Initial studies with fluorescent-labeled oligonucleotides indicate that phosphodiesters and phosphorothioates are transported actively into cells by a carrier-mediated mechanism [55]. In contrast, the more lipid soluable, uncharged methylphosphonates appear to be transported passively.

These oligonucleotide analogues were directly compared as antisense inhibitors in a CV-1 tissue culture model [56]. The cells were transfected with plasmids containing the chloramphenicol acetyltransferase gene and SV40 or HIV LTR enhancer elements. Then the cells were incubated with normal or modified oligonucleotides containing the same nucleotide sequence. The phosphorothioate analogue was about two times more effective than the methylphosphonate, which was about two times more effective than the normal oligonucleotide.

In a series of studies, Zamecnik and coworkers [57–59] compared the effects of antisense oligonucleotides with phosphodiester, methylphosphonate, and phosphorothioate linkages as inhibitors of HIV virus expression and infection in H9 or MOLT3 cells. Oligonucleotides were synthesized that were complementary to 20 different target sites within HIV RNA. The most effective inhibitors were those directed to 5′-cap or initiation sequences, and splice donor and acceptor sites. Cap or initiation sequences are necessary for ribosome assembly, while splice sites are required for accurate translation of specific proteins needed for viral function and packaging.

Oligonucleotides modified by phosphorothioate, methylphosphonate, and phorphoramidate linkages were more active than the unmodified compounds. For example, the modified ones produced 100% inhibition of syncytia formation and viral p24 synthesis at concentrations of 3 μM, while the parent phosphodiester were about half as active and rarely produced complete inhibition. Matsukura et al. [60] showed that incubation with 1 μM of a 28-nucleotide dC homopolymer with phosphorothioate linkages inhibited HIV viral synthesis in tissue culture. This effect may be related to nonspecific binding and degradation of viral RNA by RNAase H or inhibition of

HIV reverse transcriptase [61]. A follow-up study indicated that these phosphorothioate homopolymers can also inhibit DNA polymerase induced by type 1 herpes simplex virus [62].

Chronically HIV-infected H9 cells may be a more clinically relevant model. Viral protein expression was inhibited specifically by antisense phosphorothioates directed to a *trs/art* regulatory sequences or to a splice acceptor site of the virus [63, 64]. The latter paper points out that some 'random' control oligonucleotides may have sufficient RNA binding to activate RNAase H. Thus very careful computer searches are needed to maximize specificity of a phosphorothioate.

Preliminary toxicology studies in mice show no acute effects after injection of 40 mg/kg of normal and modified antisense oligonucleotides [57, 59]. Some animals died at higher doses. The mechanisms of this toxicity were not reported.

A major advantage of phosphorothioates over other oligonucleotide derivatives is their ability to be synthesized enzymatically by DNA or RNA polymerases [32]. Deoxynucleoside or nucleoside 5′-O-1-thio-triphosphates (dNTPαS or NTPαS) are incorporated into the chain as only the R_P-diastereoisomer. In contrast, chemical synthesis yields random configurations of both diastereoisomers. The enzymatically synthesized phosphorothioates are resistant to phosphodiesterases and nucleases, and have altered activity with certain restriction endonucleases. By the polymerase chain reaction it should be possible to synthesize sufficient quantities of stereospecific DNA with phosphorothioates linkages for testing as antisense inhibitors in a tissue culture system. The sulfur groups in the enzymatic products may have less steric hindrance with the target RNA helix than the chemically synthesized phosphorothioates. Thereby, the enzymatically synthesized phosphorothioates may be much more efficient.

Improved efficacy of antisense oligonucleotides may also be achieved by covalent linkage of intercalating agents to the chain [65]. Acridine derivatives were linked by a pentamethylene bridge to oligonucleotides complementary to rabbit β-globin mRNA. These derivatives are similar to those previously shown to enhance binding of oligonucleotides to double-stranded DNA [26]. The modified oligonucleotide was a more efficient inhibitor of β-globin synthesis than the unsubstituted homologue in injected Xenopus oocytes, producing 50% inhibition at 0.5 μM. The acridine alone had no effect. This improvement may be due to increased stability of the oligonucleotide-mRNA hybrid by the intercalating agent. Active groups bind with little specificity to nucleic acid sequences, so they will probably increase the nonspecific effects of the oligonucleotide.

Lower extracellular concentrations of antisense oligonucleotides may be effective if they can be transported more efficiently into cells. Lemaitre and coworkers [66] studied the effects of covalent bonding of 14,000 D polymers of L-lysine to an antisense oligonucleotide complementary to the initiation codon of a viral protein. The polycationic L-lysine may neutralize some of the negative charges on the oligonucleotide phosphate groups and allow better transport across cell membranes. This construct specifically inhibited synthesis of the viral protein in concentrations as low as 0.1 μM.

Another potential approach is to design the antisense oligonucleotide so that it will not only bind to the target mRNA sequence but also include in the duplex nucleotide sequences that can catalyze cleavage of the RNA. This idea derives from elegant experiments by Cech and colleagues [67] that showed that Tetrahymena pre-mRNA can catalyze its own cleavage and splicing without added proteins. These specific RNA sequences act like enzymes, so they are called *ribozymes*. The nucleotide sequence needed for the cleavage can be synthesized and incorporated into an antisense construct. They recently have shown that ribozymes can also cleave specific DNA sequences [68]. The advantage of this approach is that the antisense oligonucleotide can cause the cleavage of the target, dissociate, and then bind to another molecule of the mRNA or DNA, and cause its cleavage. As with other catalysts, a single molecule of antisense oligonucleotide may affect many target molecules. Investigators have transfected plasmid containing ribozyme catalytic sequences plus flanking sequences to target the RNA for a specific mRNA. High molar ratios of ribozyme to target have been needed for significant inhibition of translation [69, 70]. This weak effect is probably due to the instability of the ribozyme and its low catalytic activity. Chemical synthesis of ribozymes with some phosphorothioate linkages may increase their stability. Similar catalytic action can be achieved by covalent linkage of the oligonucleotide with EDTA-Fe(II) complexes that can cleave the target after binding [20].

For antisense chemotherapy, specific oligonucleotides must be synthesized and tested in cell-free systems, in whole cells, and finally in experimental animals. Cell-free translation systems are needed to define the optimal regions for antisense hybridization and the optimal size of the antisense oligonucleotides for each mRNA target [40]. Regions are usually sought that have minimal secondary structure and no bound proteins. Experiments with whole cells are needed to determine whether the oligonucleotide is stable in tissue culture media and cells, and whether it can be efficiently transported into the cell. Animal experiments can then define the distribution, selectivity, and toxicity of the oligonucleotides. Combination of the oligonucleotide derivatives may yield the best therapeutic agent. Other ideas include incorporation of the antisense oligonucleotide in liposomes to target them to the reticuloendothelial system and immunoconjugates to direct them to cells with specific surface receptors [30, 32]. At present the most promising combination may be to attach polylysine polymers to a phosphorothioate-linked oligonucleotide to improve cellular uptake and stability. The inhibitory effects of this complex could be further enhanced by addition of a functional group that can cleave the mRNA or intercalate with the duplex. The major problem will be to avoid nonspecific effects of the oligonucleotide analogues.

Double-stranded oligonucleotides as competitors for DNA binding factors

The rate of transcription of genes into RNA is regulated by the binding of sequence-specific nuclear proteins to regions of the DNA called *promoters* and *enhancers*. Without these binding factors, the gene under the control of a certain regulatory element will not be transcribed into mRNA, and consequently no protein will be produced. Many regulatory elements have been identified using both in vivo functional studies and in vitro binding assays. Several different nuclear proteins may bind to individual promoters and enhancers. Interaction of these factors with themselves and other transcriptional factors creates a mechanism to tightly control the expression of specific genes. The binding sites for these proteins are usually less than 12 base pairs [71, 72].

Double-stranded DNA segments or oligonucleotides containing the binding sequence for a specific nuclear factor have been shown to compete for binding of that factor to its promoter or enhancer region [73, 74]. These observations suggest a potential new approach to control the expression of a specific gene: a) the synthesis of double-stranded oligonucleotides containing the binding sequences for a specific nuclear binding factor needed for transcription of the gene; and b) transport of the double-stranded oligonucleotide into the nucleus in sufficient concentration that it binds this nuclear factor and prevents it from interacting with the promoter or enhancer for the gene. We have investigated this approach with a model system.

We showed that in vitro transcription of the adenovirus *E1B* gene can be inhibited using synthetic double-stranded oligonucleotides [75]. This gene was chosen since it contains only two nuclear factor binding sites in its promoter, a TATA box and an SP1 binding site [76]. Chemically synthesized oligonucleotides corresponding to both strands of the SP1 binding site were annealed and incubated with the *E1B* gene in a transcriptional assay system in vitro. The oligonucleotides inhibited the rate of transcription of this gene to 10% of control with a concentration less than 1 μM. In contrast, the constituent single-stranded oligonucleotides were less effective.

The use of double-stranded oligonucleotides that compete for the binding of nuclear binding factors poses unique considerations. Nuclear factor binding may be cooperative; more than one nuclear factor may need to interact for optimal transcription of the gene. Double-stranded oligonucleotides can easily be synthesized that contain more than one binding site for a nuclear factor or factors. Oligonucleotides with multiple SP1 binding sites were synthesized to address these questions. An oligonucleotide with three SP1 sites was approximately 11 times more effective that an oligonucleotide with only one SP1 site. The increased effectiveness of oligonucleotides with several SP1 sites is consistent with a recent report that this nuclear factor has non-DNA binding domains that can interact [77]. If similar interactions occur between different nuclear binding factors, oligonucleotides with two or more different binding sites may be highly selective as competitors for these binding factors. Thus, one may be able to design oligonucleotides that are selective for the binding factors needed for expression of specific genes and impart the necessary specificity. A combination of binding sites that mimics the transcriptional unit for a particular gene may allow regulation of only that gene.

Chemical modifications similar to those used for antisense oligonucleotides can be made to further enhance the effectiveness of double-stranded oligonucleotides. Phosphorothioates have been shown to form double-stranded structures, so they are the best current option [32]. We have recently shown that an oligonucleotide with two SP1 sites and phosphorothioate linkages inhibited in vitro *E1B* transcription 95% at 0.09 μM, while the corresponding normal phosphodiester required 0.69 μM for 80% inhibition.

This study has provided guidelines for producing an effective inhibitor of *E1B* transcription in vitro. Specifically, double-stranded oligonucleotides with phosphorothioate linkages and multiple nuclear factor binding sites are effective competitors for SP1 binding. Whether this approach can be used in whole cells or animal models has yet to be determined. We have recently showed that these double-standard phosphorothioate oligonucleotides can be taken up by cells and are currently studying these effects in tissue culture lines stably transfected with specific target promoters and reporter genes. What makes this approach promising is the much lower concentrations needed to achieve inhibition of expression.

A comparison of methods to control gene expression

Each of the three methods discussed to inhibit gene expression act in a unique way, and present certain advantages and disadvantages. DNA binding polymers act by binding in the minor groove of the DNA helix and, with the aid of a specific functional group, can cleave the DNA. Partial sequence specificity is achieved through selective binding to G-C- or A-T-rich regions. Further specificity can be achieved with short oligonucleotide sequences that are complementary to regions of DNA with single-stranded character or form a triple-helix structure in the major groove of DNA. Functional groups attached to these oligonucleotides can covalently link them to the DNA or cleave the DNA strand.

Antisense oligonucleotides act by sequence-specific binding to an mRNA through exact base pairing between the oligonucleotide and the mRNA sequence. Double-stranded oligonucleotides act by binding nuclear factors involved in transcription. Sequence specificity for the DNA biding region of these proteins is needed to optimally compete for the nuclear binding factor.

These three methods each act upon a different site: DNA, mRNA, or a nuclear protein. The target in least abundance is a specific segment of DNA, so direct binding of an oligonucleotide to DNA should be the most efficient. Practically, the binding may be dependent upon the generation of a replication fork to yield a single-stranded region or synthesis of an oligonucleotide that can form a triple-stranded structure.

Single DNA copies of genes are transcribed into many mRNA copies. Therefore, higher concentrations of antisense oligonucleotides may be required to interact with mRNA. The efficiency of these antisense oligonucleotides may be further decreased by regions of secondary structure in mRNA, by degradation of the oligonucleotide-RNA duplex by RNAase H, and by nonspecific binding to nucleic acid and proteins. These problems may explain the high molar ratios of antisense oligonucleotide to mRNA that are necessary for inhibition of translation.

Competing for binding of nuclear factors appears to require much lower molar ratios of oligonucleotide to target than with antisense oligonucleotides for efficient inhibition. This may be due to the low abundance of the nuclear binding factors and the regular helical structure of the short double-stranded oligonucleotides. Chemical modifications of these oligonucleotides should allow them to enter cells more efficiently and to be less susceptible to nuclease degradation. Whether a modified double-stranded oligonucleotide will be more or less efficient than a modified single-stranded oligonucleotide is not known.

Each of these approaches shows promise for an anticancer therapy. The need for further research, especially in aspects of cell delivery, is critical. Controlling gene expression with the use of oligonucleotides is a very effective method to inhibit these genes in vitro. The challenge for the next decade is to apply these methods in a clinical setting.

References

1. Bishop JM. The molecular genetics of cancer. Science 235:305–311, 1987.
2. Weinstein IB. The origins of human cancer: molecular mechanisms of carcinogenesis and their implications for cancer prevention and treatment. Cancer Res 48:4135–4143, 1988.
3. Leder A, Pattengale PK, Kuo A, Stewart TA, Leder P. Consequences of widespread deregulation of the c-myc gene in transgenic mice: multiple neoplasms and normal development. Cell 45:485–495, 1986.
4. Sinn E, Muller W, Pattengale P, Tepler I, Wallace R, and Leder P. Coexpression of MMTV/v-Ha-ras and MMTV/c-myc genes in transgenic mice: synergistic action of oncogenes *in vivo*. Cell 49:465–475, 1987.
5. Rauscher FJ, Cohen DR, Curran T, Bos TJ, Vogt PK, Bohmann D, Tjian R, and Franza BR Jr. Fos-associated protein p39 is the product of the jun proto-oncogene. Science 240:1010–1016, 1988.
6. Lippman ME, Dickson RB, Gelmann EP, Rosen N, Knabbe C, Bates S, Bronzert D, Huff K, and Kasid A. Growth regulation of human breast carcinoma occurs through regulated growth factor secretion. J Cell Biochem 35:1–16, 1987.
7. Klein G. The approaching era of the tumor suppressor genes. Science 238:1539–1545, 1987.
8. Friend SH, Bernards R, Rogelj S, Weinberg RA, Rapaport JM, Albert DM, and Dryja TP. A human DNA segment with properties of the gene that predisposes to retinoblastoma and osteosarcoma. Science 323:643–646, 1986.

9. DeCaprio JA, Ludlow JW, Figge J, Shew JY, Huang CM, Lee WH, Marsillo E, Paucha E, and Livingston DM. Large tumor antigen forms a specific complex with the product of the retinoblastoma susceptibility gene. Cell 54:275–283, 1988.
10. Laug WE and Bogenmann E. Plasminogen activator inhibitors in vascular smooth muscle cells. In: The Pharmacology and Toxicology of Proteins, JS Holcenberg and JL Winkelhake (eds). Alan R. Liss, New York, 1987, pp. 325–335.
11. Hashimoto Y and Shudo K. Drugs which interact with DNA. Molecular design of antitumor agents. Life Chem Rep 6:231–265, 1988.
12. Kopka ML, Yoon C, Goodsell D, Pjura P, and Dickerson RE. The molecular origin of DNA-drug specificity in netropsin and distamycin. Proc Natl Acad Sci USA 82:1376–1380, 1985.
13. Goodsell D and Dickerson RE. Isohelical analysis of DNA groove-binding drugs. J Med Chem 29:727–733, 1986.
14. Woynarowski, JM, McHugh, M, Sigmund, RD, and Beerman, TA. Modulation of topoisomerase II catalytic activity by DNA minor groove binding agents distamycin, Hoechst 33258, and 4′,6-diamidine-2-phenylindole. Mol Pharmacol 35:177–82, 1989.
15. McHugh, MM, Woynarowski, JM, Sigmund, RD, and Beerman, TA. Effect of minor groove binding drugs on mammalian topoisomerase I activity. Biochem Pharmacol 38: 2323–2328, 1989.
16. Dervan P. Design of sequence specific DNA-binding molecules. Science 232:464–471, 1987.
17. Krowicki K, Balzarini J, DeClercq E, Newman RA, and Lown JW. Novel DNA groove binding alkylators: design, synthesis and biological evaluation. J Med Chem 31:341–345, 1988.
18. Moy BC, Petzold GL, Badiner GJ, Kelly RC, Aristoff PA, Adams EG, Li LH, and Bhuyan BK. Characterization of B16 melanoma cells resistant to the CC-1065 analogue U-71,184. Cancer Res 50:2485–2492, 1990.
19. Kohn KW, Hartley JA, and Mattes WB. Mechanisms of DNA sequence selectivity of guanine-N7 positions by nitrogen mustards. Nucleic Acids Res 15:10531–10549, 1987.
20. Boutorin AS, Vlassov VV, Kazakov SA, Kutiavin IV, and Podyminogin MA. Complementary addressed reagents carrying EDTA-Fe(II) groups for directed cleavage of single stranded nucleic acids. FEBS Lett 172:43–46, 1984.
21. Vlassov VV, Gorn VV, Ivanova EM, Kazakov SA, and Mamaev SV. Complementary addressed modification of oligonucleotide d(pGpGpCpGpGpA) with platinum derivative of oligonucleotide d(pTpCpCpGpCpCpTpTpT). FEBS Lett 162:286–289, 1983.
22. Abramova TV, Vlassov VV, Lebedev AV, and Ryte AS. Complementary addressed modification of nuclear acids with the alkylating derivatives of oligothymidylate ethyl phosphotriesters. FEBS Lett 236:243–245, 1988.
23. Moser HE and Dervan PB. Sequence-specific cleavage of double stranded helical DNA by triple helix formation. Science 238:645–650, 1987.
24. Rajagopal P and Feigon J. NMR studies of triple-strand formation from the homopurine-homopyrimidine deoxyribonucleotides $d(GA)_4$ and $d(TC)_4$. Biochemistry 28:7859–7870, 1989.
25. Francois JC, Saison-Behmoaras T, Chassignol M, Thuong NT, and Helene C. Sequence-specific cleavage of single- and double-stranded DNA by oligonucleotides covalently linked to 1,10-phenanthroline. J Biol Chem 264:5891–5898, 1989.
26. Helene C, Monteray-Garestier T, Saison T, Takasugi M, Toulme JJ, Asseline U, Lancelot G, Maurizot JC, Toulme F, and Thuong NT. Oligonucleotides covalently linked to intercalating agents: a new class of gene regulatory substances. Biochimie 67:777–783, 1985.
27. Perrouault L, Asseline U, Rivalle C, Thoung NT, Bisagni E, Giovannangeli C, LeDuon T, and Helene C. Sequence-specific artificial photo-induced endonucleases based on triple helix-formed oligonucleotodes. Nature 344:358–360, 1990.
28. Mizuno T, Chou MY, and Inouye M. A unique mechanism regulating gene expression: translational inhibition by a complementary RNA transcript (micRNA). Proc Natl Acad

Sci USA 81:1966–1970, 1984.
29. Zamecnik PC and Stephenson ML. Inhibition of Rous sarcoma virus replication and cell transformation by a specific oligonucleotide. Proc Natl Acad Sci USA 75:280–284, 1978.
30. Oligonucleotides: antisense inhibitors of gene expression. In: Topics in Molecular and Structural Biology, JS Cohen (ed). CRC Press, Boca Raton, FL, 1989, p. 255.
31. Stein CA and Cohen JS. Oligonucleotides as inhibitors of gene expression: a review. Cancer Res 48:2659–2668, 1988.
32. Zon G. Oligonucleotide analogues as potential chemotherapeutic agents. Pharmaceutical Res 5:539–549, 1988.
33. Melton DA. Injected anti-sense RNAs specifically block messenger RNA translation *in vivo*. Proc Natl Acad Sci USA 82:144–148, 1985.
34. Rebagliati MR and Melton DA. Antisense RNA injections in fertilized frog eggs reveal an RNA duplex unwinding activity. Cell 48:599–605, 1987.
35. Izant JG and Weintraub H. Inhibition of thymidine kinase gene expression by antisense RNA: a molecular approach to genetic analysis. Cell 36:1007–1015, 1984.
36. Izant JG and Weintraub H. Constitutive and conditional suppression of exogenous and endogenous genes by antisense RNA. Science 229:345–352, 1985.
37. Kim SK and Wold BJ. Stable reduction of thymidine kinase activity in cells expressing high levels of antisense RNA. Cell 42:129–138, 1985.
38. Yokoyama K and Imamoto F. Transcriptional control of the endogenous myc proto-oncogene by antisense RNA. Proc Natl Acad Sci USA 84:7363–7367, 1987.
39. Rosenberg UB, Preiss A, Seifert E, Jackle H, and Knippie DC. Production of phenocopies by Kruppel antisense RNA injection into Drosophila embryos. Nature 313:703–706, 1985.
40. Coleman J, Hirashima A, Inokuchi Y, Green PJ, and Inouye M. A novel immune system against bacteriophage infection using complementary RNA (micRNA). Nature 315:601–603, 1985.
41. To RY, Booth SC, and Nieman PE. Inhibition of retroviral replication by anti-sense RNA. Mol Cell Biol 6:4758–4762, 1986.
42. Pestka S, Daugherty BL, Jung V, Hotta K, and Pestka RK. Anti-mRNA: specific inhibition of translation of single mRNA molecules. Proc Natl Acad Sci USA 81:7525–7528, 1984.
43. Mahler LJ and Dolnick BJ. Specific hybridization arrest of dihydrofolate reductase mRNA in vitro using anti-sense RNA or anti-sense oligonucleotides. Arch Bioch Biophys 253:214–220, 1987.
44. Shuttleworth J and Colman A. Antisense oligonucleotide-directed cleavage of mRNA in Xenopus oocytes and eggs. EMBO J 7:427–434, 1988.
45. Walder RY and Walder JA. Role of RNase H in hybrid-arrest translation by antisense oligonucleotides. Proc Natl Acad Sci USA 85:5011–5015, 1988.
46. Heikkila R, Schwab G, Wickstrom E, Loke SL, Pluznik DH, Watt R, and Neckers LM. A c-myc antisense oligonucleotide inhibits entry into S phase but not progress from G_0 to G_1. Nature 328:445–449, 1987.
47. Jaskulski D, DeRiel JK, Mercer WE, Calabretta B, and Baserga R. Inhibition of cellular proliferation by antisense oligonucleotides to PCNA cyclin. Science 240:1544–1546, 1988.
48. Miller PS, McParland KB, Jayaraman K, and Ts'o P. Biochemical and biological effects of nonionic nucleic acid methylphosphonates. Biochemistry 20:1874–1880, 1981.
49. Ts'o POP, Miller PS, and Greene JJ. Nucleic acid analogs with targeted delivery as chemotherapeutic agents. In: Development of Target-Oriented Anticancer Drugs, YC Cheng, B Goz and M Minkoff (eds). Raven Press, New York, 1983, pp. 189–206.
50. Smith C, Aurelian L, Reddy M, Miller P, and Ts'o P. Antiviral effect of an oligo(nucleoside methylphosphonate) complementary to the splice junction of herpes simplex virus type I immediate early pre-mRNAs 4 and 5. Proc Natl Acad Sci USA 83:2787–2791, 1986.
51. Kean JM, Murakami A, Balke KR, Cushman CD, and Miller PS. Photochemical cross-linking of psoralen-derivatized oligonucleotide methylphosphorates to rabbit globin messenger RNA. Biochemistry 27:9113–9121, 1988.

52. Kulka M, Smith CC, Aurelian L, Fishelevich R, Meade K, Miller P and Ts'o POP. Site specificity of the inhibitory effects of oligo (nucleoside methylphosphonates) complementary to the acceptor splice junction of herpes simplex virus type 1 immediate early mRNA 4. Proc Natl Acad Sci USA 86:6868–6872, 1989.
53. Vasanthakumar G and Ahmed NK. Modulation of drug resistance in a daunorubicin resistant subline with oligonucleotide methylphosphonates. Cancer Commun 1:225–232, 1989.
54. User Bulletin. Applied Biosystems Separation Systems 44:1–18, 1987.
55. Loke SL, Stein CA, Zhang XH, Mori K, Nakanishi M, Subasinghe C, Cohn JS, and Neckers LM. Characterization of oligonucleotide transport into living cells. Proc Natl Acad Sci USA 86:3474–3478, 1989.
56. Marcus-Sekura CJ, Woerner AM, Shinozuka K, Zon G, and Quinnan J. Comparative inhibition of chloroamphenicol acetyltransferase gene expression by antisense oligonucleotide analogues having alkyl phosphotriester, methylphosphonate and phosphorothioate linkages. Nucleic Acids Res 15:5749–5763, 1987.
57. Goodchild J, Agrawal S, Civeira MP, Sarin PS, Sun DX, and Zamecnik PC. Inhibition of human immunodeficiency virus replication by antisense oligodeoxynucleotides. Proc Natl Acad Sci USA 85:5507–5511, 1988.
58. Sarin PS, Agrawal S, Civiera MP, Goodchild J, Ikeuchi T, and Zamecnik PC. Inhibition of acquired immunodeficiency syndrome virus by oligo-deoxynucleoside methylphosphonates. Proc Natl Acad Sci USA 85:7448–7451, 1988.
59. Agrawal S, Goodchild J, Cibiera MP, Thornton AH, Sarin PS, and Zamecnik PC. Oligodeoxynucleoside phosphoramidates and phosphorothioates as inhibitors of human immunodeficiency virus. Proc Natl Acad Sci USA 85:7079–7083, 1988.
60. Matsukura M, Shinozuka K, Zon G, Mitsuya H, Teitz M, Cohen JS, and Broder S. Phosphorothioate analogs of oligonucleotides: Inhibitors of replication and cytopathic effects of human immunodeficiency virus. Proc Natl Acad Sci USA 84:7706–7710, 1987.
61. Majundar C, Stein CA, Cohen JS, Broder S, and Wilson SH. Step wise mechanism of HIV reverse transcriptase: primer function of phosphorothioate oligonucleotide. Biochemistry 28:1340–1346, 1989.
62. Gao W, Stein CA, Cohen JS, Outschman GE, and Cheng YC. Effect of phosphorothioate homo-deoxynucleotides on herpes simplex virus type 2-induced DNA polymerase. J Biol Chem 264:11521–11526, 1989.
63. Matsukura M, Zon G, Shinozuka K, Robert-Guroff M, Shimada T, Stein CA, Mitsuya H, Wong-Staal F, Cohen JS, and Broder S. Regulation of viral expression of HIV *in vitro* by an antisense phosphorothioate oligo-deoxynucleotide against rev (art/trs) in chronically infected cells. Proc Natl Acad Sci USA 86:4244–4248, 1989.
64. Agawal S, Ikeuchi T, Sun D, Sarin PS, Konopka A, Maizedl J, and Zamecnik PC. Inhibition of human immunodeficiency virus in early infected and chronically infected cells by antisense oligonucleotide and their phophorothioate analoque. Proc Natl Acad Sci USA 86:7790–7794, 1989.
65. Cazenave C, Loreau N, Thuong NT, Toulme JJ, and Helene C. Enzymatic amplification of translation of rabbit β-globin mRNA mediated by antimessenger oligonucleotides covalently linked to intercalating agents. Nucleic Acids Res 15:4717–4736, 1987.
66. Lemaitre M, Bayard B, and Lebleu B. Specific antiviral activity of a poly(L-lysine)-conjugated oligodeoxyribonucleotide sequence complementary to vesicular stomatitis virus N protein mRNA initiation site. Proc Natl Acad Sci USA 84:648–652, 1987.
67. Been MD and Cech TR. One binding site determines sequence specificity of tetrahymena pre-rRNA self-splicing, trans-splicing and RNA enzyme activity. Proc Natl Acad Sci USA 47:207–216, 1987.
68. Herschlag D and Cech TR. DNA cleavage catalysed by the ribozyme from Tetrahymena. Nature 344:405–409, 1990.
69. Cameron FH and Jennings PA. Specific gene suppression by engineered ribozyme in monkey cells. Proc Natl Acad Sci USA 86:9139–9143, 1989.

70. Chang PS, Cantin EM, Zaia JA, Ladne PA, Stephens DA, Sarver N, and Ross JJ. Ribozyme-mediated site-specific cleavage of the HIV-1 genome. Clin Biotechnol 2:23–31, 1990.
71. Gidoni D, Dynan WS, and Tjian R. Multiple specific contacts between a mammalian transcription factor and its cognate promoters. Nature 312:409–413, 1984.
72. McKnight SL and Kingsbury R. Transcriptional control signals of a eukaryotic protein-coding gene. Science 217:316–324, 1982.
73. Singh HR, Sen D, Baltimore D, and Sharp PA. A nuclear factor that binds to a conserved sequence motif in transcriptional control elements of immunoglobulin genes. Nature 314: 154–158, 1986.
74. Davison BL, Egly JM, Mulvihill ER, and Chambon P. Formation of stable preinitiation complexes between eukaryotic class B transcription factors and promoter sequences. Nature 301:680–686, 1983.
75. Wu H, Holcenberg JS, Tomich J, Chen J, Jones PA, Huang SH, and Calame KL. Inhibition of *in vitro* transcription by specific double-stranded oligonucleotides. Gene 89:203–209, 1990.
76. Wu L, Rosser DSE, Schmidt MC, and Berk A. A TATA box implicated in EIA transcription activation of a simple adenovirus 2 promoter. Nature 326:512–515, 1987.
77. Kadonaga JT, Courey AJ, Ladika J, and Tjian R. Distinct regions of Sp1 modulate binding and transcriptional activation. Science 242:1566–1570, 1988.

2. Modulation of the activity of cancer chemotherapeutic agents by dipyridamole

Rakesh Goel and Stephen B. Howell

Introduction

Dipyridamole (2,6,-bis-diethanolamino-4,8-dipiperidinopyrimido-5,4-d-pyrimidine) is a pyrimidopyrimidine derivative (illustrated in figure 1) that is commonly prescribed as a coronory vasodilator for the long-term therapy of angina pectoris, as an antiplatelet drug in various thrombotic disorders, such as coronory and cerebrovascular disease [1, 2]. However, only its therapeutic use in combination with coumarin anticoagulants to reduce the risk of postoperative thromboembolic complications in patients undergoing cardiac valve replacement is approved by the Food and Drug Administration [3]. Dipyridamole can modulate the activity of a number of chemotherapeutic agents and may have the ability to enhance their therapeutic index. We review here the cellular and biochemical mechanisms by which dipyridamole alters cancer cell sensitivity and point out potential clinical applications.

Preclinical pharmacology of dipyridamole

The mechanism by which dipyridamole inhibits aggregration has been reviewed recently [1]. Dipyridamole appears to interfere with platelet function by at least two mechanisms. First, it inhibits cAMP-dependent phosphodiesterase, resulting in an increase in intraplatelet cyclic AMP and subsequent potentiation of the platelet-inhibiting actions of prostacyclin, leading to direct stimulation of the release of prostacyclin by vascular endothelium. Second, it also inhibits cellular uptake and metabolism of adenosine, thereby increasing the adenosine concentration at the platelet-vascular interface. Adenosine is a potent vasodilator and the coronory vasodilatory action of dipyridamole probably results from its ability to inhibit cellular adenosine uptake and metabolism, thereby allowing the accumulation of adenosine in plasma [2].

Nucleoside transport in mammalian cells is complex [1, 4–5]. The cellular uptake of nucleosides occurs by at least four transport systems [4], as well as by simple diffusion [1]. One or more of these mechanisms may be opera-

Franco M. Muggia (ed.), NEW DRUGS, CONCEPTS AND RESULTS IN CANCER CHEMOTHERAPY.

Kluwer Academic Publishers, Boston. *ISBN 0-7923-1253-8*

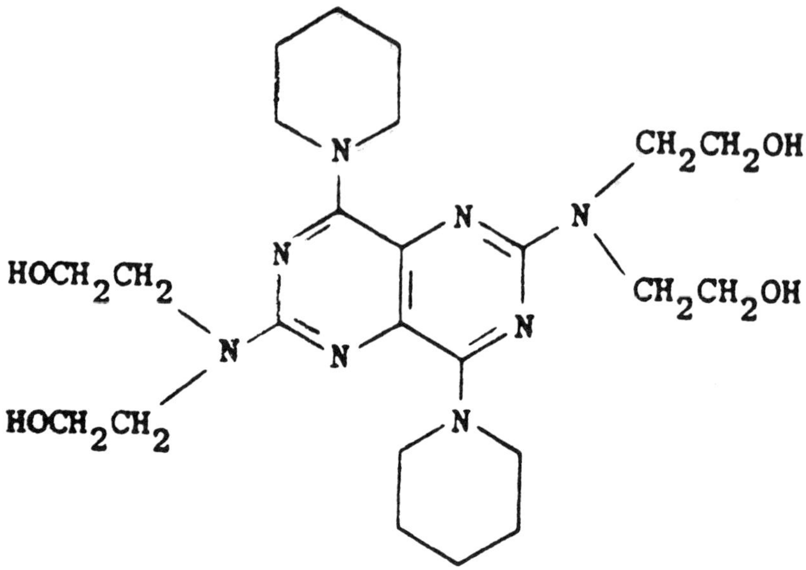

Figure 1. The chemical structure of dipyridamole.

tional in a given cell type. Two equilibrative (facilitated diffusion) transporters have been distinguished based upon their sensitivity to the nucleoside analog nitrobenzylthioinosine (NBMPR) [4–5]. The NBMPR-sensitive transporter has a high-affinity binding site for the nucleoside (K_D = 0.1–1.0 nM), and occupancy of this site by this agent correlates with inhibition of nucleoside transport. The NBMPR-insensitive transporter lacks the high-affinity site for the nucleoside and is not inhibited by NBMPR at concentrations up to 1 μM. Both transporter systems have wide substrate specificity, accepting both ribonucleosides and deoxyribonucleosides of the physiological purine and pyrimidine bases, as well as numerous cytotoxic nucleosides.

Two energy-dependent concentrative nucleoside transport systems also exist [5, 6]. These systems require in inward sodium gradient and are not sensitive to NBMPR. These transporters have much narrower substrate specificity than the equilibrative systems.

Dipyridamole can interfere with the NBMPR-sensitive nucleoside transporter by a competitive process [5]. This inhibition by dipyridamole is at a different site on the transporter than that by NBMPR. Dipyridamole appears to also inhibit the NBMPR-insensitive transporter [6], although its effect on the other two transporters has not yet been reported.

The ability of dipyridamole to inhibit facilitated nucleoside transport across cell membranes has been demonstrated in a broad range of malignant cell lines by many researchers. Kessel et al. [7] were among the first to make this observation when they showed that dipyridamole can inhibit the uptake of adenosine and deoxycytidine in L1210 cells. Paterson et al. [8]

showed that dipyridamole inhibited the transport of uridine into HeLa cells and also observed that dipyridamole protected cells against the cytotoxic action of cytosine arabinoside, adenosine arabinoside, and other toxic nucleosides by inhibiting their cellular uptake.

Weber et al. [9], in a review of their previous experiments, found that dipyridamole alone can be cytotoxic to cancer cells. It can block the uptake of several purine and pyrimidine nucleosides into log-phase hepatoma 3924A cells. The LD_{50} for dipyridamole in a 7-day clonogenic assay was 20 μM. Dose-response experiments showed that 10–75 μM dipyridamole inhibited the incorporation of uridine and thymidine into the DNA and RNA of these cells. The inhibition of DNA and RNA biosynthesis was attributed, in part at least, to inhibition of the transport of salvage precursors. The cell kill was 76% upon exposure to 60–100 μM dipyridamole, and the corresponding nucleotide levels were at most 50% of control. Weber et al. raised the possibility that dipyridamole interfered with the biochemical commitment of hepatoma cells by unbalancing the pools of nucleotide triphosphates.

As described in Weber's review [9], there is substantial clinical evidence that marked inhibition of the *de novo* pathways of nucleotide biosynthesis by antimetabolites often fails to produce significant cytotoxicity. This resistance can result from the marked increases in the activities of the enzymes of the purine and pyrimidine salvage pathways, causing a repletion of intracellular nucleotide pools. Dipyridamole, by blocking the cellular uptake of nucleosides, can enhance the cytotoxic action of these antimetabolites and can overcome this type of resistance.

Most solid tumors, such as gastrointestinal and gynecologic malignancies, are slow growing, and the majority of their cells are in the resting phase of the cell cycle. Zhen et al. [10] showed that hepatoma 3924A cells in stationary phase were insensitive to the inhibitory action of 10 μM dipyridamole on nucleoside transport, whereas proliferating cells are relatively sensitive to dipyridamole. These results suggested that dipyridamole may be unable to modulate the activities of antimetabolites in slowly growing tumors. They found that mitomycin C, and particularly amphotericin B, were capable of restoring the sensitivity of nonproliferating cells to dipyridamole, suggesting that a drug such as amphotericin must be used with dipyridamole to maximize the latter's synergy with antimetabolites against tumors with low growth fractions.

It appears that dipyridamole can be cytotoxic to hematologic cell lines, as well as to solid-tumor cell lines. Farmer et al. [11] showed that 3 μM dipyridamole was cytotoxic to L1210 cells. Hirose et al. [12] showed that the growth of myeloperoxidase-positive nonlymphoid cell lines was strongly inhibited by 18 μM dipyridamole, whereas other hematologic cell lines were resistant to the growth-inhibiting effects of dipyridamole. These differences were not related to variations in inhibition of nucleoside uptake in the cell lines, as the inhibition of radiolabeled thymidine uptake was identical in all of them.

Batista et al. [13] and Mamytbekova et al. [14] explored the possibility that dipyridamole affected the formation of metastases. They rationalized that since platelet aggregation may be involved in the metastatic spread of tumors, then dipyridamole might inhibit the formation or the growth of metastases. Mamytbekova et al. [14] did not observe any inhibitory effect of dipyridamole on the development of metastases from subcutaneously implanted Lewis lung carcinomas in mice. However, flurbiprofen, another antiplatelet agent, did significantly reduce the number of metastases that developed. Batista et al. [13] examined the effects of dipyridamole on the human tumor SKNMC neuroblastoma and U87MG glioblastoma cell lines. Both cell lines can activate platelet aggregation. Tumor cell growth was inhibited by at least 70% upon exposure to 5 μM dipyridamole, cellular nucleoside uptake was significantly inhibited by 1 μM dipyridamole, and the platelet-activating ability of the SKNMC cell line was inhibited significantly by 2.5 μM dipyridamole (the U87MG cell line's platelet-aggregating activity was only modestly reduced by 10 μM dipyridamole). These results suggest that dipyridamole can potentially inhibit the growth of tumor metastases, but whether this occurs by affecting tumor cell metabolism due to a reduction in cellular nucleoside incorporation, by suppressing the tumor's ability to activate platelets, or by some other mechanism that has not yet been defined is unknown. Since therapeutic doses of dipyridamole result in plasma concentrations of about 3.5 μM [15], dipyridamole may be useful in some circumstances as an antimetastatic agent.

Cornwell et al. [16, 17] suggested that dipyridamole may have opposite effects on cell growth and metastases. Dipyridamole functions as an antioxidant, thus stimulating the prostanoid pathways and inhibiting the peroxide pathways of fatty acid metabolism. They showed in their experiments that dipyridamole caused a proliferation of smooth muscle cells in vitro via these mechanisms, concluding that dipyridamole is a growth factor and an ineffective antimetastatic agent.

In their recent review, Grem and Fischer [5] commented on the immunologic actions of dipyridamole as one potential mechanism of its modulation of other drugs. They reported on experiments in which dipyridamole has been found to induce interferon production in vitro and in mice. In addition, they stated that dipyridamole has also been reported to have some antiviral activity. However, Havlin et al. [18] recently observed that neither low-dose dipyridamole (150 mg orally or 10-mg intravenous bolus) increased interferon levels 24 hours after administration in normal volunteers, nor did high-dose dipyridamole (7.7–13 mg/kg by continuous intravenous infusion per 24 hours for 72 hours) increase steady-state levels in patients with metastatic cancer. The changes in the interferon levels of patients who have normal immune function who are given high-dose interferon must still be determined.

Newell et al. [19] studied the effects of intravenous infusions of dipyridamole on tritiated thymidine incorporation into the DNA of bone marrow, gastrointestinal tract epithelium, and an ascitic form of the Walker carcinoma in Wistar rats. A 40 mg/kg injection of dipyridamole reduced thymidine incorporation into DNA of bone marrow and gastrointestinal tract epithelium to 25% control, and produced peak dipyridamole plasma levels of 10–15 μM. A 100 mg/kg intravenous injection of dipyridamole produced peritoneal concentrations above 20 μM. However, dipyridamole at these concentrations had no effect on nucleoside uptake or survival of the tumor cells, suggesting that the resistance was due to an intrinsic property of the tumor cells, rather than to the pharmacokinetic properties of the drug. Moyer et al. [20] showed that a 100 mg/kg injection of dipyridamole did not significantly reduce the salvage of uridine by liver or kidney in mice, while only a small and short-lived decrease in uridine salvage in both subcutaneously and intraperitoneally implanted L1210 cells was observed. Belt and Noel [21] later showed that 10 μM dipyridamole in serum-free buffer inhibited thymidine uptake in Walker cells. Dipyridamole is 97% protein bound in the rat plasma [15] and at least 99% protein-bound in human plasma [5, 15, 22]. In a review of other investigators' experiments, Newell et al. [19] indicated that dipyridamole concentrations of up to 1 μM were necessary to maximally inhibit the cellular uptake or incorporation of nucleosides in serum-free medium. Therefore, these data suggest that the plasma levels of pharmacologically active free dipyridamole in animal plasma were too low to alter nucleoside uptake in at least tumor cells and that the concentrations that can be achieved in human plasma by conventional oral doses of dipyridamole [15] would be too low to modulate the activity of drugs against normal or tumor tissue.

Methotrexate and dipyridamole

Methotrexate is an antimetabolite that exerts its action primarily through inhibition of the enzyme dihydrofolate reductase (DHFR) [23, 24]. This enzyme maintains the intracellular pool of reduced folates (figure 2). Reduced folates (tetrahydrofolates) are essential cofactors needed for the transfer of one-carbon units in a number of biosynthetic reactions. The *de novo* synthesis of the purine precursor inosinic acid, the pyrimidine thymidine, and ultimately DNA and RNA are dependent upon the intracellular concentrations of reduced folates. Methotrexate may also directly inhibit *de novo* purine synthesis [25].

Methotrexate inhibits DHFR, resulting in the accumulation of cellular folates in the inactive, oxidized form and a cessation first of thymidine and then of purine synthesis. An excess of non-protein-bound drug is necessary to inhibit nucleotide synthesis because of the reversible nature of methotrexate binding to DHFR. In cells, both naturally occurring folates and methotrexate are conjugated with glutamic acid to form polyglutamyl derivatives. The long-chain polyglutamyl derivatives of methotrexate bind to

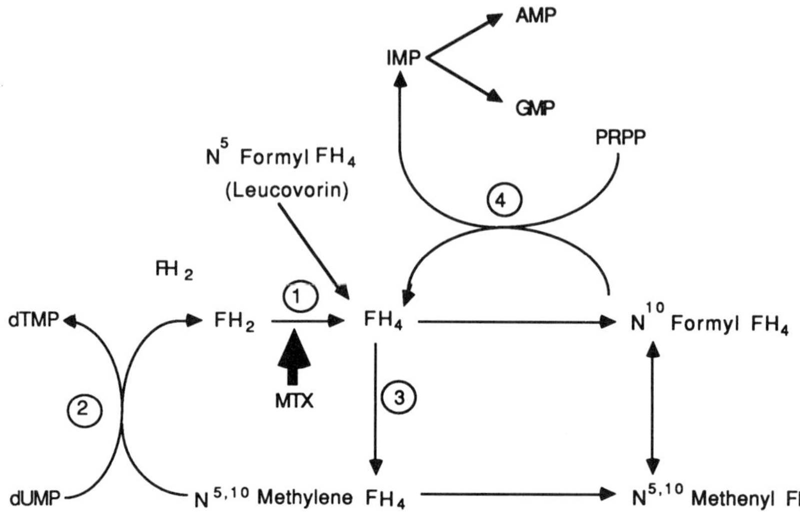

Figure 2. The sites of methotrexate activity in the cellular metabolic pathyways. FH_2 = dihydrofolate; FH_4 = tetrahydrofolate; PRPP = 5-phosphoribosyl-1-pyrophosphte; IMP = inosine monophosphate; AMP = adenosine monophosphate; GMP = guanosine monophosphate; dUMP = deoxyuridine monophosphate; dTMP = deoxythymidine monophosphate. Enzymes: 1, dihydrofolate reductase; 2, thymidylate synthase; 3, serine hydroxymethyl transferase; 4, glycinamide ribotide transformylase/amino-imidazole carboxamide ribotide transformylase. The thick arrow represents enzyme inhibition.

DHFR at least as strongly as parent drug, but they disassociate less easily from DHFR than parent drug. The polyglutamyl derivatives are retained by cells, with half-lives of retention increasing with increasing glutamyl chain length.

Dipyridamole increases the cytotoxicity of methotrexate, in part by decreasing uptake and salvage of nucleosides. Investigators have found this interaction to take place in vitro with Chinese hamster ovary (CHO) cells and three human osteogenic sarcoma cell lines [26], ascitic sarcoma 180 cells [27], L1210 cells [28], and human colonic carcinoma HCT 116 cells [29]. Dipyridamole, at concentrations ranging from 3 to 10 μM, significantly reduced the incorporation and salvage of thymidine in these cells. This resulted in further depletion of intracellular dTTP pools and therefore further impairment of DNA synthesis, causing increased cell death.

Kennedy et al. [30] found another mechanism by which dipyridamole modulates methotrexate activity in the human breast carcinoma MDA.MB.436 cell line. Dipyridamole increased the accumulation of methotrexate in these cells, largely by increasing the relative intracellular amount of long-chain polyglutamyl (7–10 glutamate residues) methotrexate derivatives. As these derivatives of methotrexate disassociate from DHFR less easily, and efflux from the cell more slowly than other methotrexate species, they account for a relatively large amount of the toxicity contributed by methotrexate. Cabral et al. [27] also found that dipyridamole could decrease the efflux of intracellular methotrexate. However, as Ackland and Schilsky state in their review [24], the 1 hour incubation with both drugs is probably too short for significant polyglutamation of methotrexate to take place, implying that dipyridamole was inhibiting methotrexate efflux through some other mechanism in Cabral's experiments.

The above experiments [28, 29] also showed that tissue culture medium, supplemented with either nucleosides or undialyzed serum, can partially counteract the interaction of dipyridamole with methotrexate. In humans, the plasma concentrations of nucleosides and hypoxanthine are about as high (i.e., 0.1–1.0 μM for nucleosides and 0.2–64 μM for hypoxanthine [28]) as those found in tissue culture medium supplemented with 8% fetal bovine serum (i.e., 0.6 μM for thymidine and 9 μM for hypoxanthine [29]). This may provide one mechanism of resistance to methotrexate. Only continuous parenteral infusions of dipyridamole have achieved the 5–10 μM plasma concentrations of total drug that are necessary to block the salvage of these concentrations of nucleosides by cells in vitro [5, 31, 32]. However, it is likely that much higher concentrations of dipyridamole are needed to provide sufficient levels of pharmacologically active free drug for this effect to take place in vivo.

Different cell lines may have different mechanisms of nucleoside transport and different amounts of salvage enzyme activity, and thus the modulation of methotrexate by dipyridamole would be expected to vary from line to line [29]. This heterogeneity could be an advantage if nucleoside transport in normal cells, such as bone marrow, were less sensitive to the inhibitory effects of dipyridamole than tumor cells. On the other hand, if normal cells were at least as sensitive to dipyridamole's effects on nucleoside salvage as tumor cells, then this two-drug combination would have a low therapeutic index and it would not be of much clinical value [26, 33].

The ability of dipyridamole to selectively increase the toxicity of methotrexate against tumor cells, and thereby to increase its therapeutic index, has been tested in several phase I/pharmacologic trials. Subar et al. [34] conducted a phase I study giving dipyridamole at a dose of 50–75 mg orally every 6 hours, and escalating the duration of methotrexate given at 2.5 mg twice a day from 2 to 3 days. Dipyridamole was continued for 4 days beyond the termination of methotrexate administration. Courses were repeated every 3 weeks. The dose-limiting toxicities, reached when methotrexate was administered for 6–5 days, were mucosal and hematologic. They concluded that dipyridamole enhanced the toxicity of this methotrexate regimen, as it is usually nontoxic [34, 35]. Some antitumor responses were seen. This group [35] later performed a phase II study to test the efficacy of this regimen against colorectal carcinoma. A similar pattern of toxicity was seen as in the phase I study, with no significant response rate. The plasma dipyridamole concentrations ranged from 1 to 4 μM. They had shown [27] that dipyridamole at concentrations ranging from 3 to 10 μM were necessary to prevent salvage of nucleosides in vitro. Therefore, they felt that the plasma concentrations of dipyridamole were not sufficient for a sustained period of time to produce a significant therapeutic effect. In addition, the greater protein levels in plasma compared to tissue culture medium would be expected to result in much lower pharmacologically active non-protein-bound dipyridamole concentrations in plasma compared to tissue culture medium supplemented with fetal calf serum. The dose of oral dipyridamole required to achieve an effective concentration would be too toxic, and therefore it was felt that only parenteral infusions of dipyridamole could effectively enhance methotrexate's antitumor effect.

Other phase I/pharmacokinetic studies have been performed [31, 36, 37]. Dipyridamole and methotrexate have been given in various oral and parenteral schedules. Plasma dipyridamole levels ranging from 2.7 to 11.4 μM were noted with oral dosing [36, 37], and a mean steady-state total and free dipyridamole level of 5.5 ± 0.26 (SD) μM and 20.1 ± 1.4 nM with continuous intravenous infusion [31]. The dose-limiting toxicities were mucositis and myelosuppression. Dipyridamole significantly increased the toxicity of methotrexate only when dipyridamole was given by continuous intravenous infusion [31]. In this case, dipyridamole did not affect the pharmacokinetics of methotrexate. Only in one study were a few responses observed with this drug combination [36]. These studies suggested that clinically significant biochemical modulation of methotrexate by dipyridamole, as evidenced by the systemic toxicity, was achievable by continuous intravenous infusion of dipyridamole. However, the antitumor effect in these trials was generally quite disappointing.

A major problem with the drug regimens mentioned above has been their narrow therapeutic indexes. One approach to improving the selectivity of drugs is to deliver them directly to the environment of the tumor so that total drug exposure there is much larger than in normal tissues. Intraperitoneal administration of drug to tumors confined to the peritoneal cavity is one example of this concept [38].

We have recently tested this concept by conducting a phase I/pharmacokinetic study by administering methotrexate and dipyridamole together at high concentrations intraperitoneally by long-duration continuous infusion [39]. We hypothesized that a prolonged infusion of methotrexate (a cell-cycle phase-specific drug), and the synergy afforded by high concentrations of dipyridamole, would produce a selective increase in the activity of methotrexate in the peritoneal cavity without enhancing its systemic toxicity.

Initially, 2.16 mg/m^2/day methotrexate and 12 mg/m^2/day dipyridamole were delivered together as a constant intraperitoneal infusion for 48 hours. With dose escalation, eventually 4.32 mg/m^2/day methotrexate, with the same initial daily dose of dipyridamole, were administered for 168 hours. Forty-seven courses were administered to 18 patients. The mean steady-state peritoneal and plasma methotrexate concentrations, at the higher dose level, were 7.80 and 0.11 μM, respectively (figure 3). The total (protein-

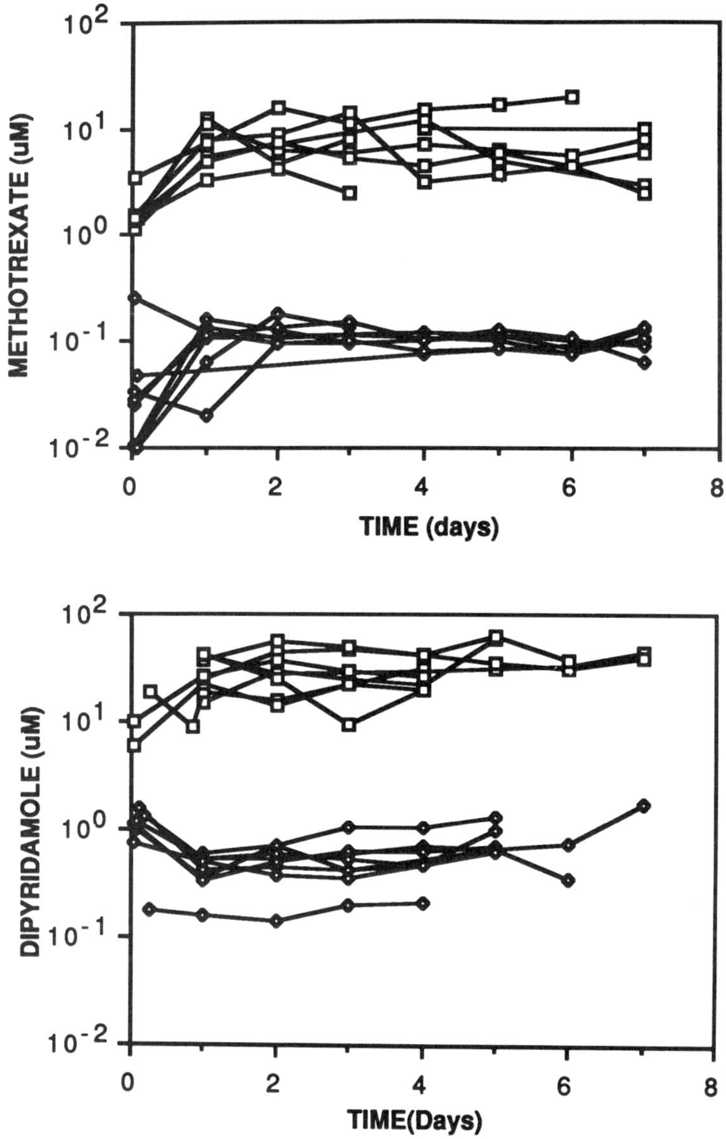

Figure 3. The peritoneal (squares) or plasma (diamonds) concentrations of methotrexate (top panel) and dipyridamole (bottom panel) after the bolus intraperitoneal administration of 0.90 mg methotrexate and 10.1 mg dipyridamole followed by a daily infusion of 4.32 mg/m^2 methotrexate and 12 mg/m^2 dipyridamole. (Reproduced by permission from J Clin Oncol 7:262–269, 1989.)

bound and free) dipyridamole levels in these two compartments were 30.3 and 0.57 μM (figure 3). The mean free non-protein-bound dipyridamole concentrations in the peritoneal cavity and in the plasma were 11.74 μM and below the detection limit of 0.005 μM, respectively. Chemical peritonitis was the dose-limiting toxicity. Of 13 patients evaluable for response, three had a minor response (two with ovarian carcinoma and one with colonic carcinoma).

This study demonstrated that the concentrations of dipyridamole in the peritoneal cavity were in the range that produces synergy with methotrexate, whereas the concentrations of both drugs in the systemic circulation were too low for a significant interaction to take place. Future phase II and III studies need to be conducted to determine whether the purported synergy is taking place and whether this approach can improve response rates and survival.

Fluoropyrimidines and dipyridamole

5-fluorouracil (5FU) has at least two biochemical metabolites that may be responsible for its cytotoxicity [23, 40]. It is first converted to the nucleotide fluorouridine monophophate (FUMP) (figure 4). This nucleotide may be further converted to two active metabolites, fluorouridine 5′-monophosphate (FUTP) and 5-fluoro-2′deoxyuridine-5′monophosphate (FdUMP). FUTP is

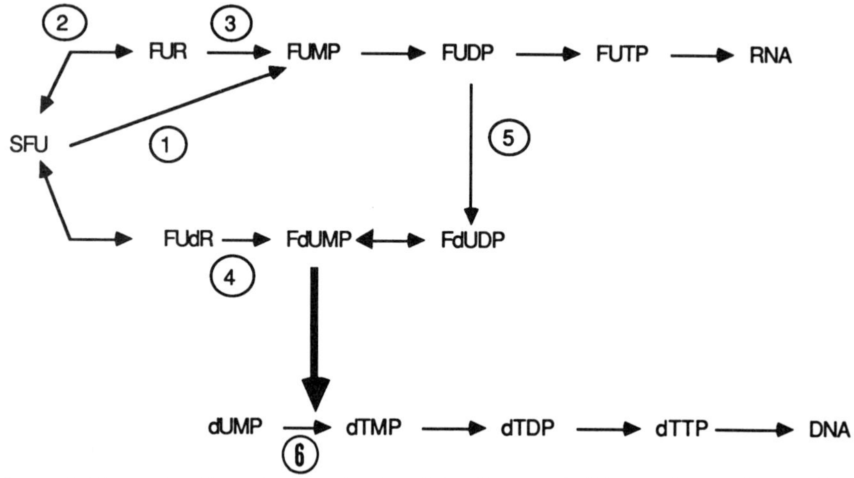

Figure 4. The metabolic pathways of intracellular fluoropyrimidines. FUR = fluorouridine; FUMP = fluorouridine monophosphate; FUDP = fluorouridine diphosphate; FUTP = fluorouridine triphosphate; FUdR = fluorodeoxyuridine; FdUMP = fluorodeoxyuridine monophosphate; FdUDP = fluorodeoxyuridine triphosphate; dUMP = deoxyuridine monophosphate; dTMP = deoxythymidine monophosphate; dTDP = deoxythymidine diphosphate; dTTP = deoxyuridine triphosphate. Enzymes: 1, orotic acid phosphoribosyl transferase; 2, uridine phosphorylase; 3, uridine kinase; 4, thymidylate kinase; 5, ribonucleoside diphosphate reductase; 6, thymidylate synthase. The thick arrow represents enzyme inhibition.

incorporated into RNA and inhibits mRNA processing and stability. FUTP may also be incorporated into DNA. Errors in repair of this latter lesion may cause cell death. FdUMP forms a ternary complex with reduced folate and thymidylate synthase (thymidylate synthetase) and inhibits the eventual formation of dTTP, one of the precursors of DNA. 5-fluoro-2′deoxyuridine (FUdR) is converted to FdUMP by a nucleoside kinase and primarily inhibits thymidylate synthase, with lesser effects on RNA than 5FU.

Resistance to 5FU may develop through the decreased activities of enzymes required to convert 5FU to active metabolites. Another mechanism of resistance may be an increase in thymidylate synthase concentration or activity. Other potential means by which cells may protect themselves against the cytotoxicity of fluoropyrimidines include the salvage of preformed nucleosides. However, the extent to which tumor cell utilization of salvage pathways is important in circumventing 5FU toxicity is not well defined. Specifically, if 5FU cytotoxicity is due to its inhibition of thymidylate synthase, then circulating levels of thymidine may be may be capable of partially repleting intracellular dTTP pools. Dipyridamole, by inhibiting nucleoside transport, may prevent this nucleoside salvage and augment 5FU toxicity.

Dipyridamole has been found to increase the cytotoxicity of 5FU in the human colon carcinoma HCT 116 cell line [5, 41–43], human epidermoid carcinoma Hep-2 and human breast cancer MCF-7 lines [37], and (when combined with the uridine phosphyrylase inhibitor, benzylacyclouridine) human colon carcinoma CT38 cell line [44]. This modulation was dose and time dependent [5, 41–43]. For example, the cell number after a 72-hour exposure to 5 μM 5FU and 5 μM dipyridamole was 22% of that seen with 5FU alone. Since almost 90% of the effect was produced by 0.5 μM dipyridamole, this concentration was used for subsequent experiments.

The interaction was related to a selective increase in FdUMP levels resulting from blockage of FUdR efflux and increased deoxyribose-1-phosphate (dR-1-P) pools due to decreased deoxyuridine efflux. Dipyridamole did not significantly alter the total amount of 5FU that was incorporated into either DNA or RNA, nor did it affect the natural ribonucleotide pool sizes. The reduction of FUdR efflux resulted in an increase in its conversion to FdUMP. Deoxyuridine increased FdUMP levels by serving as a donor of a dR-1-P moiety to generate FUdR from 5FU. Grem and Fischer [5] suggested that in cancer cells that can significantly catabolize FdUMP, the ability of dipyridamole to block the efflux of FUdR and to increase the deoxyribose-1-phosphate pools may provide an effective means of selectively increasing FdUMP levels and increasing 5FU toxicity. Dipyridamole has also been found to inhibit the uptake of fluorouridine and FUdR in these cells, but it did not affect the uptake of 5FU.

Recent experimental findings by Lonn et al. [45] confirm the mechanism of augmentation of fluoropyrimidine cytotoxicity by dipyridamole. They found that dipyridamole increased the ability of both 5FU and FUdR to induce DNA fragmentation and subsequent cytotoxicity in human colon adenocarcinoma WiDr cells. They observed that dipyridamole induced defects in DNA repair by depleting cellular dTTP pools; dipyridamole did not accentuate the incorporation of the fluoropyrimidines into DNA.

It would seem logical that increasing intracellular FdUMP levels would lead to a decrease in the activity of thymidylate synthase, causing a depletion in dTTP pools. Although 5 μM 5FU decreased the activity of this enzyme in HCT 116 cells to 15–25% of control levels after 24 hours of exposure [5], the dTTP pools are virtually unchanged at the end of this time interval, with or without the further addition of 0.5 μM dipyridamole [5]. Thus, the data suggest that the depletion of dTTP pools was not the primary mechanism of 5FU toxicity in these cells and that the increase of 5FU toxicity caused by dipyridamole was not due to a further depletion of dTTP.

Although dipyridamole did significantly impair the uptake of thymidine and uridine [5, 41–43], this was not the crucial mechanism by which dipyridamole increased its cytotoxicity against HCT 116 cells. Grem and Fischer [5] suggested that in cell lines in which inhibition of thymidylate synthase is growth limiting at relatively low concentrations of fluoropyrimidines, dipyridamole can increase their cytotoxicity by this mechanism. This was the mechanism by which dipyridamole increased the cytotoxicity of 5FU in HT 29 cells [46]. Nevertheless, this potentiation of 5FU effect by dipyridamole in HCT 116 cells was overcome by a high concentration (25 μM) of thymidine, which appears to rescue cells by decreasing FdUMP formation. In addition to bypassing thymidylate synthase inhibition [43], thymidine expands the intracellular dTTP pools, which decreases the activity of thymidine kinase by feedback inhibition, resulting in decreased formation of FdUMP from FUdR.

At least one clinical study testing the interaction between 5FU and dipyridamole has been reported [5, 47]. The maximal tolerated dose of 5FU, when administered simultaneously with 7.7 mg/kg/day dipyridamole as a continuous 3-day infusion, was 3600 mg/m^2/day. 5FU was subsequently given to patients at this dose without concurrent dipyridamole to evaluate the contribution of dipyridamole to the toxicity produced by 5FU alone. The mean total and free dipyridamole levels in the plasma were 6.7 μM and 24.1 nM, respectively. The mean 5FU plasma concentrations seemed to be significantly greater, and the mean total body 5FU clearances were significantly lower when 5FU was given concurrently with dipyridamole. (The dose-limiting toxicity was stomatitis.) Dipyridamole neither increased 5FU-induced myelosuppression nor stomatitis. Two partial responses in 47 patients were seen. Preclinical data indicate that dipyridamole enhances 5 FU-induced cytotoxicity. Since tumor cells may be more susceptible to impairement of nucleoside transport than normal cells, the enhanced cytotoxicity of dipyridamole may be selective. Therefore, further clinical studies to assess this drug combination are warranted.

Several studies [46, 48–51] have been conducted with the combination of 5FU, folinic acid (leucovorin), and dipyridamole. Folinic acid can potentiate 5FU activity by stabilizing the FdUMP-thymidylate synthase complex [reviewed in 40]. Miller et al. [46] showed that dipyridamole increased the growth inhibition of human colon carcinoma HCT 116 and HT 29 cells by the 5FU/folinic acid combination. It appeared that dipyridamole was able to increase the cytotoxicity of the two-drug combination by decreasing the cellular salvage of thymidine. In four clinical studies [48–51], parenteral folinic acid and 5FU were given with concurrent oral administration of dipyridamole. The dose-limiting toxicity was oral mucositis, although some gastrointestinal toxicity, cardiac toxicity, myelosuppression, and headaches were also seen. Some responses were seen in three of the studies [48, 50], including a few patients who had failed prior 5FU and folinic acid therapy. In one study, five of thirteen patients with breast carcinoma responded [48]. These investigators suggested that thymidine salvage may be overcoming the activity of the 5FU/folinic acid combination, and the addition of the dipyridamole may produce some additional antitumor activity [49–51]. Migeod et al. [51] did not find that dipyridamole increased the toxicity of the 5FU/folinic acid combination, nor were there any responses in patients who received the three-drug combination after failing the initial 5FU/folinic acid combination.

Buzaid et al. [52] tested the ability of dipyridamole to increase the activity of FUdR in vivo and in vitro. The cytotoxicity of FUdR was increased by a median of 33.5-fold against 6 of 8 human colon carcinoma cell lines by 0.05 μM dipyridamole. Significant interaction was also seen between the two drugs against human bone-marrow colony forming units. Dipyridamole's mode of activity was thought to be mainly by inhibition of thymidine salvage and FUdR efflux. These results led to the conduct of a phase II trial of continuous intravenous infusion of FUdR (0.1 mg/kg/day for 14 days) and dipyridamole (75 mg orally five times a day for 14 days) in patients with colorectal carcinoma with metastases to the liver. Toxicities were mild and consisted mainly of mild mucositis and diarrhea. Four partial responses in 27 patients evaluable for response were observed. Seeger et al. [53] conducted a phase II trial administering oral dipyridamole (200 mg/day) and FUdR by hepatic arterial infusion (400 mg for 2 weeks every 4 weeks) to a group of similar patients. Serum dipyridamole levels were 1.2 μM, greater than 50 times that needed for in vitro FUdR uptake inhibition. At the time of their report, no significant toxicity had occurred, and dipyridamole seemed to be reducing the hepatic toxicity of hepatic artery infusion of FUdR. Three of four patients evaluable for response had achieved a partial response. These two studies suggest that the combination of FUdR and dipyridamole is well tolerated, but further trials have to be conducted to assess the contribution of dipyridamole to the response and toxicity of this two-drug regimen.

Cytosine arabinoside and dipyridamole

Cytosine arabinoside (cytarabine, ara-C) is a drug that is transported into the cell via a facilitated diffusion transport system [23]. Inside the cell it is either catabolized to the inactive metabolite ara-U or anabolized by deoxy-

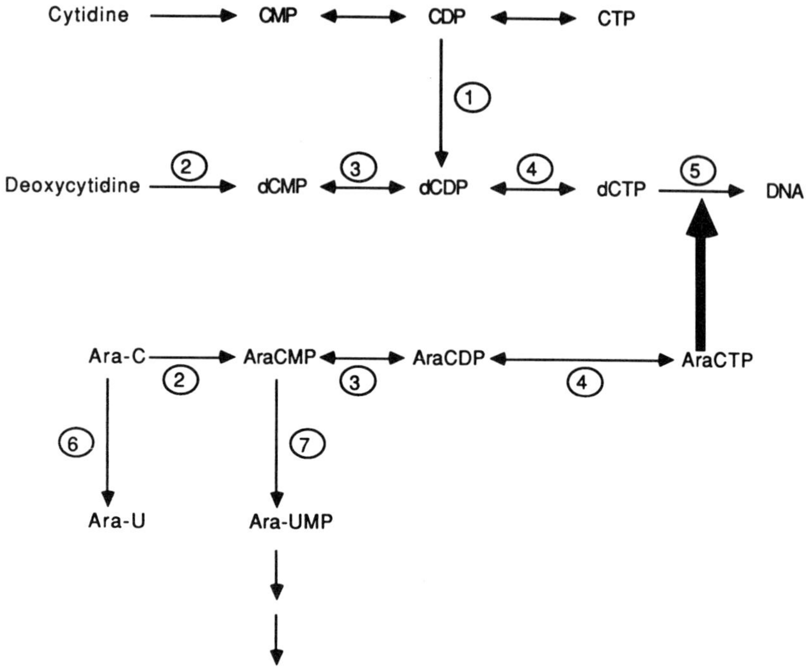

Figure 5. The metabolic pathways of cytosine arabinoside (Ara-C). (d)CMP = (deoxy)cytosine monophosphate; (d)CDP = (deoxy)cytosine diphosphate; (d)CTP = (deoxy)cytosine triphosphate; Ara-U = uracil arabinoside; AraCMP = cytosine monophosphate arabinoside; Ara-UMP = uridine monophosphate arabinoside; Ara-UTP = uridine triphosphate arabinoside; AraCDP = cytosine diphosphate arabinoside; AraCTP = cytosine triphosphate arabinoside; Enzymes: 1, ribonucleoside diphosphate reductase; 2, deoxycytidine kinase; 3, dCMP kinase; 4, nucleoside diphosphate kinase; 5, DNA polymerase; 6, cytidine deaminase; 7, dCMP deaminase. The thick arrow represents enzyme inhibition.

cytidine kinase to ara-CMP (figure 5). Although this latter reaction has been conventionally felt to be the rate-limiting step of ara-C metabolism and subsequent toxicity [23], recent evidence indicates that ara-C influx may be the rate-limiting step in some cells [54]. Ara-CMP is further metabolized to ara-CTP, the cytotoxic form of the drug. Ara-CTP competes with dCTP for DNA polymerase and is incorporated into DNA, where it blocks the further elongation of the DNA strand. The cytotoxicity of ara-C is proportional to the concentration and duration of exposure of DNA to ara-CTP.

Dipyridamole can inhibit both the influx and the efflux of ara-C by interfering with its transport. King et al. [55] studied the relative effects of dipyridamole on the uptake and the toxicity of ara-C on normal and malignant cells. They reasoned that if dipyridamole selectively inhibited the uptake of ara-C in normal tissues, then one could significantly increase the dose of ara-C that patients could safely tolerate. Murine L1210 cells, human promyelocytic HL-60 cells, and bone marrow cells from volunteers were studied. Unfortunately, they found that dipyridamole, at concentrations achievable in humans, produced at least a 90% reduction of uptake of ara-C in all three cell lines. Dipyridamole reduced the growth-inhibitory effects of ara-C on HL-60 cells in culture and protected mice from the toxic dose of this antimetabolite. Kubota et al. [56] observed a similar effect of dipyridamole on the uptake and the cytoxicity of ara-C in human T lymphoblastoid Molt 4 and HL-60 cell lines.

King et al. [55] did not find any increase in selectivity of ara-C when using dipyridamole in vitro. However, they reasoned that systemically delivered dipyridamole may allow an increase in the dose of ara-C that could be safely delivered intraperitoneally to patients with tumors confined to the peritoneal cavity. Systemic dipyridamole could reduce systemic bone marrow toxicity, while producing little if any interference with intraperitoneal antineoplastic activity. This concept has not yet been tested clinically.

Yang et al. [57] and Chan [58] demonstrated that dipyridamole can enhance the cytotoxic effect of ara-C by impairing its efflux from cells. Yang studied this phenomenon in murine leukemia L5178Y cells and Chan studied it in human ovarian carcinoma OV 2008 and human promyelocytic HL60 cells. They both observed that the sequential administration of dipyridamole after ara-C potentiated the cytotoxicity of ara-C to the cells, and this was associated with an increased retention of ara-CTP. These data suggest that by appropriate scheduling of both drugs one might permit ara-C to get into cells and then block its efflux with dipyridamole. Yang et al. [57] are evaluating the effects of dipyridamole on the cellular pharmacokinetics of ara-C in blasts from patients with acute leukemia to determine the potential therapeutic utility of this pharmacologic strategy.

Acivicin and dipyridamole

The biochemical pharmacology of acivicin has been recently reviewed [59]. It is an antimetabolite that inhibits several enzymes that are important for purine and pyrimidine metabolism. It produces increases in cellular UTP concentration, and decreases in CTP and GTP concentrations, with no alteration in ATP or ITP pools. Acivicin enters cells by a carrier-mediated transport system, which is distinct from that of the nucleosides. However, exogenous nucleosides can reverse the biochemical effects of acivicin in vitro. Dipyridamole can modulate the cytotoxicity of acivicin by interfering with this reversal.

Zhen et al. [60] found that dipyridamole inhibited the incorporation of several different nucleosides in rat hepatoma 3924A cells with a 50% inhibitory concentration of 0.5 μM. The nucleosides protected these cells from the growth-inhibitory and cytotoxic actions of acivicin. The addition of dipyridamole to culture medium containing acivicin and nucleosides could produce the same cytotoxicity to these cells as acivicin alone. Fischer et al. [61] performed similar experiments in human colon cancer VACO 5 cells and confirmed the modulatory activity of dipyridamole on acivicin.

Fischer et al. [5, 32, 62] initiated a phase I trial to test the modulation of these two drugs in humans. Simultaneous 72-hour intravenous infusions of both drugs were given to patients with advanced malignancies. The total acivicin dose was 20 mg/m^2/day, and the dipyridamole dose was escalated until the maximal tolerated dose of 7.7 mg/kg/day was reached. The peripheral infusion of dipyridamole was associated with venous irritation, thus requiring administration via a central venous catheter. The dose-limiting toxicities were headache and diarrhea, and were felt to be caused by dipyridamole. Dipyridamole did not seem to potentiate the myelosuppressive or neurotoxic toxicities of acivicin.

The relative lack of toxicity characteristic of acivicin suggested that nucleotide biosynthesis was not inhibited by dipyridamole. However, the mean steady-state total and free dipyridamole concentrations were 11.3 μM and 28 nM, respectively [5], levels sufficient to potentiate the biochemical and cytotoxic actions against human colon cancer cell lines in vitro [61]. Significant inhibition of CTP synthetase and GMP synthetase activity was evident in the lymphocytes obtained from patients while on therapy, but there was no significant decrease in the ribonucleoside triphosphate pools. This inability of dipyridamole to augment acivicin effects may have been due to insufficient inhibition of *de novo* nucleoside synthesis pathways by acivicin, the lack of importance of nucleoside salvage in the action of acivicin, or an incorrect schedule of administration of both drugs. Therefore, this lack of a consistent, pronounced effect of acivicin on *de novo* nucleotide biosynthesis precludes analysis of the role of salvage in modulating the toxicity in vivo, even though pharmacologically active plasma dipyridamole levels were achieved [36].

PALA and dipyridamole

N-phosphonacetyl-L-aspartic acid (PALA) is an analog of the transition-state intermediate of aspartate transcarbamylase [63], the second enzyme of *de novo* pyrimidine synthesis [64]. As reviewed by Markman et al. [65], this agent has shown cytoxicity to slow-growing murine tumors, such as Lewis lung carcinoma and B16 melanoma, but it is less toxic to rapidly growing murine leukemias. Most clinical trials have failed to reveal any significant antitumor activity of this agent. Markman et al. [65] postulated that the lack of activity of this drug against human tumors may be due to salvage of exogenous pyrimidine nucleosides in vivo, which would bypass the metabolic block produced by PALA. It was hypothesized that dipyridamole may inhibit the uptake of these nucleosides and increase the cytotoxicity of PALA.

The first group of experiments by this laboratory group [66] were done to assess the cytotoxicity of the drug combination against human colon carcinoma T-219, human melanoma T-242, HL-60, and normal bone marrow

(CFU-GM) cells in clonogenic assays. At 1 μM, dipyridamole increased the cytotoxicity of PALA against these cells in clonogenic assays, although concentrations of only 0.1 μM were sufficient to produce a 50% inhibition of uridine uptake. Dipyridamole also reduced the LD_{50} of PALA by 50% in mice. A similar pattern of modulation was found in OV 2008 cells [67]. The mechanism of synergy was related to the inhibition of pyrimidine salvage, resulting in lower intracellular pools of UTP and CTP, via the blockade of uridine uptake.

Markman et al. [65] (and alluded to by Chan et al. [68]) conducted a phase I trial assessing the combination of dipyridamole at 50 mg/m^2 orally every 6 hours starting 1 week before the administration of PALA and continuing for the duration of the study, and of PALA administered intravenously at escalating doses from 500 mg/m^2 to 4500 mg/m^2. They found that the maximal tolerated dose of PALA when given with dipyridamole was 80% of that when PALA was given alone. The dose-limiting toxicities were diarrhea and abdominal pain, side effects usually associated with PALA. The response rate was not significantly different from that of PALA alone; however, an encouraging response rate with soft-tissue sarcoma was observed, and they felt that a phase II study testing this drug combination against these tumors was warranted.

Chan et al. [68] found that the plasma uridine level decreased from a mean of 3.49 μM to a mean of 2.46 μM after 1 week of dipyridamole administration. PALA further reduced the uridine level 7 hours after administration to a mean of 0.87 μM. These results suggested that dipyridamole worked in synergy with PALA to lower circulating uridine levels in cancer patients by inhibiting the cellular nucleoside efflux. As the liver is the major source of uridine in the systemic circulation, dipyridamole may inhibit the release of this nucleoside from this organ. They suggested that the ability of dipyridamole to reduce the plasma pool may limit the availability of salvage metabolites and be another mechanism by which dipyridamole potentiates the activity of anticancer drugs. Moyer et al. [20] injected 100 mg/kg dipyridamole intravenously into mice. They did not find that dipyridamole significantly changed the clearance of radiolabeled uridine.

Cisplatin and dipyridamole

Cisplatin is a drug whose mechanism of cellular entry and exit are not well understood. Its cytotoxicity is related to its ability to form intrastrand and interstrand cross-links in DNA [23]. Howell et al. [69] tested the combination of both drugs on a human ovarian carcinoma OV 2008 cell line and a resistant subline. Dipyridamole significantly increased the cytotoxicity of cisplatin to these cells in a concentration dependent manner over a concentration range of 1–20 μM. The accumulation of cisplatin in both cell lines was increased to 150% of control when 20 μM dipyridamole was added (figure 6). This synergy was not significantly dependent upon blockade of

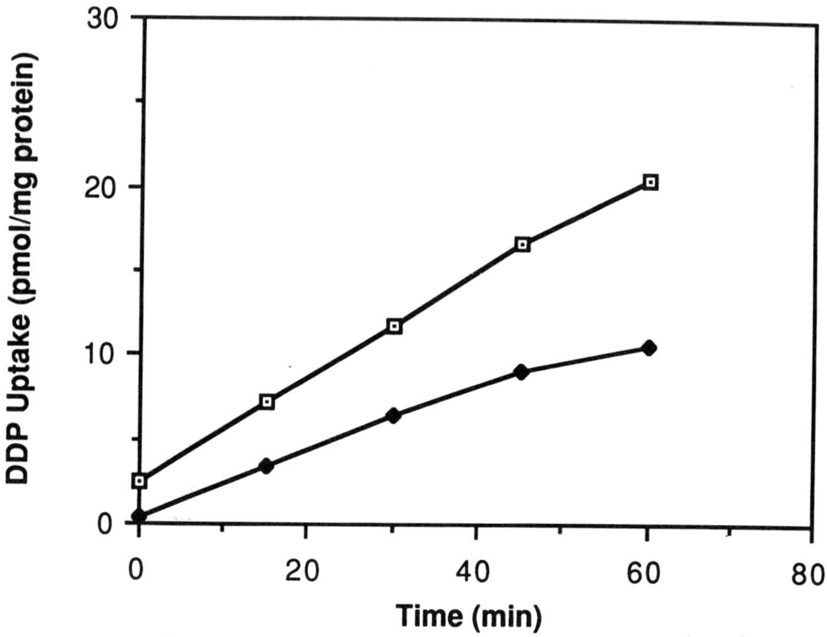

Figure 6. Cisplatin (DDP) uptake as a function of time in OV 2008 cells in the presence (open squares) or absence (closed diamonds) of 20 μM dipyridamole. (Reproduced by permission from *Biochemical Modulation of Cisplatin*, M Nicolini (ed). Martinus Nijhoff, Norwell, MA, 1987).

NBMPR-inhibitable nucleoside transport alone, nor was it due to a decrease of cisplatin efflux, nor to an increase in the intracellular concentration of cyclic AMP. The maximal modulation of cisplatin activity took place at dipyridamole concentrations of 20 μM, which are much higher than those obtained with oral dosing of dipyridamole [15, 22]. Concentrations of 5–10 μM can be achieved in the plasma by continuous parenteral infusion [5, 31, 32], and concentrations of at least 100 μM can be achieved in the peritoneal cavity by intraperitoneal instillation [39]. It would be warranted to test this two-drug combination in these two circumstances.

Etoposide, doxorubicin, or Vinca alkaloids and dipyridamole

Howell et al. [70, 71] studied the ability of dipyridamole to modulate the cytotoxicity of etoposide (VP-16), doxorubicin (Adriamycin®), and vinblastine to OV 2008 cells. Dipyridamole interacted synergistically with etoposide in clonogenic assays [70]. A 5.5-fold reduction in the IC_{50} of these cells was observed when they were incubated with 20 μM dipyridamole. Dipyridamole increased the cellular content of etoposide in a concentration-dependent

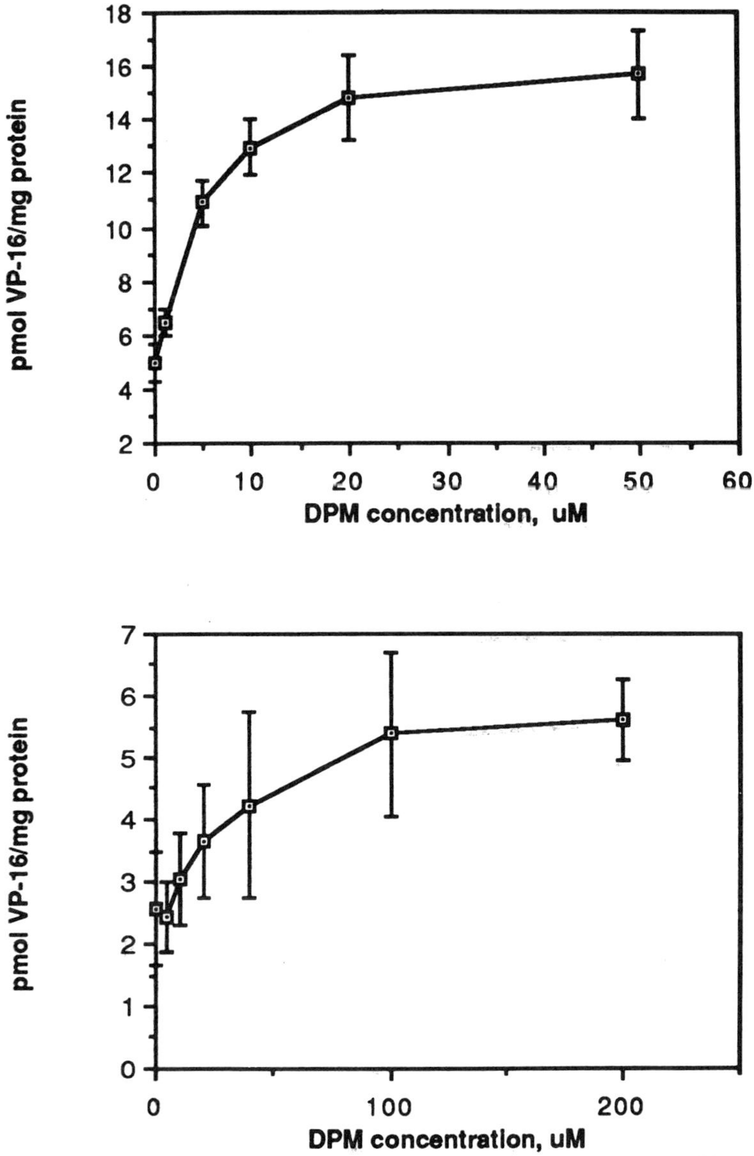

Figure 7. Steady-state cellular etoposide (VP-16) content as a function of dipyridamole concentration. Human ovarian carcinoma OV 2008 cells were exposed simultaneously to 1 μM [^{3}H]-VP-16 and an increasing concentration of dipyridamole for 1 hour. Upper panel, calls incubated in RPMI 1640 containing 10% fetal calf serum. Lower panel, cells incubated in undiluted human plasma. Each point represent the mean of three separate experiments, with each experiment performed using duplicate cultures. Vertical lines indicate standard deviation. (Reproduced by permission from Cancer Res 70:4147–4153, 1989.)

manner; 10 μM dipyridamole increased the cellular etoposide pools by just over two-fold (figure 7A). In human plasma, a 10-fold higher concentration of dipyridamole was needed to produced the same degree of modulation due to extensive protein binding of both drugs (figure 7B). Dipyridamole modulated the activity of etoposide in part by inhibiting its efflux.

Howell et al. [71] also found that dipyridamole interacted synergistically with both doxorobicin and vinblastine against OV 2008 cells. They found that dipyridamole inhibited the initial efflux of all three drugs, and in addition, dipyridamole significantly augmented the initial influx of vinblastine. However, there was no correlation between the extent of efflux inhibition and the magnitude of the dipyridamole-induced increase in cellular content, indicating that dipyridamole was modulating these three drugs through additional mechanisms. They suggested that dipyridamole may potentiate the activity of many drugs participating in the multiple drug resistance phenotype. Others have also demonstrated the interaction of dipyridamole with Vinca alkaloids and doxorubicin. Hirose et al. [72] tested the effect of dipyridamole on the activity of vincristine and several other drugs against three human cell lines, the human T-cell lymphablastoid leukemia line MOLT-3, Burkitt's lymphoma line BL-TH, and acute myelocytic leukemia line ML-1. Dipyridamole inhibited the growth of these cells lines with the IC_{50} values ranging from 14.3 to 27.2 μM. Together, vincristine and dipyridamole had synergistic inhibitory effects on the growth of these cell lines. At concentrations up to 10–20 μM, dipyridamole enhanced the intracellular accumulation of vincristine in a dose-dependent manner. Inhibition of vincristine efflux from cells was the apparent mechanism of this interaction. Kusumoto et al. [73] found that dipyridamole increased the cytotoxicity of doxorubicin against HeLa cells. Dipyridamole also potentiated the growth inhibition of doxorubicin against Sarcoma 180 cells and improved the effect of doxorubicin on the increase in lifespan of Sarcoma 180 tumor-bearing mice. The authors attributed the modulation to an increase in the association of doxorubicin with DNA resulting from an increase in cellular accumulation, as opposed to inhibition of efflux, although the initial influx was not measured. Yin et al. [74] also showed that dipyridamole increased the cytotoxicity of doxurubicin in doxorubicin-resistant P388 leukemia cells. This was due to an increase in accumulation, rather than an increase in intracellular retention of the anthracycline. The efflux of doxorubicin was minimally affected by dipyridamole in these cells. Dipyridamole also increased doxorubicin-induced DNA single-strand breaks, but did not inhibit DNA repair.

The total dipyridamole concentrations required for modulation of etoposide, Vinca alkaloids, and doxorubicin by dipyridamole are within the range attainable by parenteral [37] or intraperitoneal administration [39]. Thus, clinical trials to determine whether dipyridamole can enhance the therapeutic index of drugs that participate in the multiple drug resistance phenotype are feasible and should be performed.

Other drugs and dipyridamole

Several investigators [75, 76] have studied the interaction of dipyridamole with CB3717, an antifolate inhibitor of thymidylate synthase, in vitro. They found that dipyridamole potentiated the activity of this antimetabolite. The mechanisms of cell death from CB3717 with and without dipyridamole were analyzed. CB3713 resulted in intracellular accumulation of dUTP, leading to uracil misincorporation in DNA, its subsequent excision, and finally DNA strand breakage. Dipyridamole enhanced dUTP accumulation (and thereby potentiated the cytotoxicity of CB3717) by inhibiting deoxyoridine efflux and by inhibiting thymidine uptake (which results in depletion of dTTP pools, ultimately resulting in a further accumulation of dUTP).

Kung et al. [77] found that dipyridamole enhanced the toxicity of the 2′-deoxyadenosine and deoxycoformycin combination against L1210 cells. The latter two drugs increase the intracellular levels of dATP, which is the cytotoxic metabolite in these cells. It appears that dipyridamole inhibits the efflux of catabolites of this nucleotide.

Janowska-Wieczorek et al. [78] showed that dipyridamole and other nucleoside inhibitors can selectively decrease the toxicity of tubericidin, a cytotoxic nucleoside, against normal bone marrow cells compared to human leukemia HL-60 and K562 cells lines by impairing its efflux.

Conclusions

Dipyridamole can modulate the activity of a wide range of important chemotherapeutic agents by a variety of mechanisms. The main mechanisms include an alteration of the cellular transport of nucleosides and a change in the cellular accumulation of the drugs themselves.

It is likely that only continuous parenteral infusions of dipyridamole produce plasma concentrations consistently high enough for modulation of drug activity to take place. It appears that these plasma dipyridamole levels are sufficient to modulate the activity of antimetabolites via alterations in the cellular transport of nucleosides, but it is unclear whether these dipyridamole levels are high enough to increase the activity of other drugs, including those participating in the multiple drug resistance phenotype.

The p-glycoprotein that is associated with the multiple drug resistance phenotype has been found in the capillary endothelial cells at the brain-brain barrier site [79]. If the protein is involved in restricting entry of common chemotherapeutic agents into the brain, and if dipyridamole is found to impair the activity of this protein, then dipyridamole may be useful in potentiating the activity of systemic chemotherapy against brain tumors.

The ideal modulating agent is one that selectively increases the activity of chemotherapeutic agents against tumor cells, but not normal cells. However, in the clinical trials conducted up to the present time, there is little convincing evidence that dipyridamole has significantly increased the therapeutic index of any chemotherapeutic agent.

One way that the therapeutic index of a dipyridamole/chemotherapy drug regimen can be improved is through the use of regional treatments. Examples of these treatments include intracavitary (i.e., intraperitoneal, intrapleural, intrapericardial, intrathecal) and intraarterial treatments. The concentrations of both dipyridamole and chemotherapeutic drugs can be maintained in the vicinity of the tumor at high concentrations, potentially causing significant tumor kill; the concentrations of these agents in the plasma compartment would be much lower, thereby minimizing systemic toxicity. In addition, the greater degree of protein binding of drugs in plasma compared to the region of the drug administration would lead to a further increase in the selectivity of the drugs. This pattern of selective activity was achieved in the phase I trial of intraperitoneal methotrexate and dipyridamole that has already been described [35]. The high peritoneal levels of both drugs contributed to the observed responses and the peritoneal dose-limiting toxicity; the relatively minimal systemic side effects were attributed to the low plasma levels of both drugs.

Additionally, the therapeutic index of chemotherapeutic drugs could be increased by dipyridamole through its ability to nonselectively impair the cellular uptake of certain drugs. As previously described, dipyridamole does inhibit the cellular uptake of ara-C in tumor and normal cells [46]. This lack of selectivity could be put to advantage through the use of regional treatment. If ara-C was injected regionally, and dipyridamole was injected intravenously, then potential systemic toxicity would be minimized without significant impairment of regional antitumor activity.

There is a need for more laboratory studies to more fully determine the mechanisms of modulation of chemotherapy drugs by dipyridamole and for more clinical studies to test these concepts. The putative modulation of various chemotherapy drugs by dipyridamole must also be shown to take place in vivo, as well as in vitro. With the exploitation of further discoveries, one might be able to design effective chemotherapeutic regimens using dipyridamole, and ultimately, dipyridamole might become as important in cancer treatment as many chemotherapeutic agents are today.

Acknowledgments

We would like to thank Seema Goel for drawing figures 2, 4, and 5. This work was supported by the Alberta Heritage Trust Fund for Medical Research, and it was conducted in part by the Clayton Foundation for Research —California Division. Dr. Howell is a Clayton Foundation investigator.

References

1. Fitzgerald GA. Dipyridamole. N Engl J Med 316:1247–1257, 1987.
2. Dawicki DD, Agarwal KC, and Parks RE Jr. Adenosine metabolism in human whole blood. Effects of nucleoside transport inhibitors and phosphate concentration. Biochem Pharmacol 37:621–626, 1988.
3. Meyer GF. Dipyridamole, drugs for human use; drug efficacy study implementation, and revocation of exemption, followup notice, and opportunity for hearing. Fed Reg 52: 1662–1668, 1987.
4. Vijayalakshmi D and Belt JA. Sodium-dependent nucleoside transport in mouse intestinal epithelial cells. J Biol Chem 263:19419–19423, 1988.
5. Grem JL and Fischer PH. Enhancement of 5-fluorouracil anticancer activity by dipyridamole. Pharmac Ther 40:349–379, 1989.
6. Crawford CR, and Belt JA. Sodium-dependent, concentrative nucleoside transport in Walker 256 rat carcinosarcoma cells. Biochem Biophy Res Commun 175:846–851, 1991.
7. Kessel D and Dodd DC. Effects of persantin on several transport systems of murine leukemias. Biochim Biophys Acta 288:190–194, 1972.
8. Paterson ARP, Kolassa N, and Cass CE. Transport of nucleoside drugs in animal cells. Pharmacol Ther 12:515–536, 1981.
9. Weber G, Jayaram HN, Pillwein K, Natsumeda Y, Reardon MA, and Zhen Y-S. Salvage pathways as targets of chemotherapy. Adv Enzyme Regul 26:335–352, 1987.
10. Zhen Y-S, Reardon MA, and Weber G. Amphotericin B renders stationary phase hepatoma cells sensitive to dipyridamole. Biochem Biophys Res Commun 140:434–439, 1986.
11. Farmer JL and Prager MD. Inhibition of lymphoproliferation by dipyridamole. Biochem Pharmacol 31:1381–1386, 1982.
12. Hirose M, Takeda E, Ninimiya T, Kuroda Y, and Miyao M. Inhibitory effect of dipyridamole on the growth of various human hematologic cell lines. Tokushima J Exp Med 33:51–57, 1987.
13. Batista E, del Prado J, Almirall L, Jamieson GA, and Ordinas A. Inhibitory effects of dipyridamole on growth, nucleoside incorporation, and platelet-activating capability in the U87MG and SKNMC human tumor cell lines. Cancer Res 45:4048–4052, 1985.
14. Mamytbekova A, Rezabek K, Kacerovska H, Grimova J, and Svobodova. Antimetastatic effect of flurbiprofen and other platelet aggregation inhibitors. Neoplasma 33:417–421, 1986.
15. Mahoney C, Wolfram KM, Cochetto DM, and Bjornsson TD. Dipyridamole kinetics. Clin Pharmacol Ther 31:330–338, 1982.
16. Cornwell DG, Lindsey JA, Zhang H, and Morisaki N. Fatty acid metabolism and cell proliferation. VI. Properties of antithrombotic agents that influence metastasis, In: Icosanoids and Cancer, H Thaler-Dao (ed). Raven Press, New York, 1984, pp. 205–222.
17. Cornwell DG and Morisaki N, Fatty acid paradoxes in the control of cell proliferation: prostaglandins, lipid peroxides, and cooxidation reactions. In: Free Radicals in Biology (Vol. 6), WA Pryor (ed). Academic Press, New York, 1984, pp. 95–147.
18. Havlin KA, Inglot AD, Willson JKV, Borden EC, Grossberg S, Szulc B, Gladysz A, and Groehlich B. Lack of interferon production by dipyridamole. J Interferon Res 8:135–136, 1988.
19. Newell DR, O'Connor PM, Calvert AH, and Harrap, KR. The effect of the nucleoside transport inhibitor dipyridamole on the incorporation of [^{3}H]thymidine in the rat. Biochem Pharmacol 35:3871–3877, 1986.
20. Moyer JD, Malinowski N, and Cysyk RL. The effect of 3-deazauridine and dipyridamole on uridine utilization by mice. Eur J Cancer Clin Oncol 22:323–327, 1986.
21. Belt JA and Noel LD. Nucleoside transport in Walker 256 rat carcinosarcoma and S49 mouse lymphoma cells. Differences in sensitivity to nitrobenzylthioinosine and thiol reagents. Biochem J 232:681–688, 1985.

22. Bjornsson TD and Mahoney C. Pharmacokinetics of dipyridamole. Thromb Res Suppl. IV:93–104, 1983.
23. Chabner BA and Myers CE. Clinical pharmacology of cancer chemotherapy. In: Cancer Principles and Practice of Oncology, VD DeVita, S Hellman, and SA Rosenberg (eds). J.B. Lippincott, Philadelphia, 1989, pp. 349–395.
24. Ackland SP and Schilsky RL. High-dose methotrexate: a critical reappraisal. J Clin Oncol 5:2017–2031, 1987.
25. Allegra CJ, Hoang K, Yeh GC, Drake JC, and Baram J. Evidence for direct inhibition of de novo purine synthesis in human MCF-7 breast cells as a principal mode of metabolic inhibition by methotrexate. J Biol Chem 262:13520–13526, 1987.
26. Nelson JA and Drake S. Potentiation of methotrexate toxicity by dipyridamole. Cancer Res 44:2493–2496, 1984.
27. Cabral S, Leis S, Bover L, Nembrot M, and Mordoh J. Dipyridamole inhibits reversion by thymidine of methotrexate effect and increases drug uptake in Sarcoma 180 cells. Proc Natl Acad Sci USA 81:3200–3203, 1984.
28. Muggia FM, Slowiaczek P, and Tattersall MHN. Characterization of conditions in which dipyridamole enhances methotrexate toxicity in L1210 cells. Anticancer Res 7:161–166, 1987.
29. Van Mouwerik TJ, Pangallo CA, Willson JKV, and Fischer PH. Augmentation of methotrexate cytotoxicity in human colon cancer cells achieved through inhibition of thymidine salvage by dipyridamole. Biochem Pharmacol 36:809–814, 1987.
30. Kennedy DG, van den Berg HW, Clarke R, and Murphy RF. Enhancement of methotrexate cytotoxicity towards the MDA.MB.436 human breast cancer cell line by dipyridamole. Biochem Pharmacol 35:3053–3056, 1986.
31. Willson JKV, Fischer PH, Remick SC, Tutsch KD, Grem JL, Nieting L, Alberti D, Bruggink J, and Trump DL. Methotrexate and dipyridamole combination chemotherapy based upon inhibition of nucleoside salvage in humans. Cancer Res 49:1866–1870, 1989.
32. Willson JKV, Fischer PH, Tutsch K, Alberti D, Simon K, Hamilton RD, Bruggink J, Koeller JM, Tormey DC, Earhart RH, Ranhosky A, and Trump DL. Phase I clinical trial of a combination of dipyridamole and acivicin based upon inhibition of nucleoside salvage. Cancer Res 48:5585–5580, 1988.
33. Lee MW and Chan CH. Potentiation of methotrexate (MTX) and 5-FU effect on human cancer and normal bone marrow cells by dipyridamole (DIP). Proc Am Assoc Cancer Res 28:410, 1987.
34. Subar M, Muggia F, Green MD, and Fischer P. Phase I study of daily oral methotrexate with concurrent dipyridamole (DP) for inhibition of salvage pathway 'rescue'. Proc Am Soc Clin Oncol 5:42, 1987.
35. Wadler S, Subar M, Green MD, Wiernik PH, and Muggia FM. Phase II trial of oral methotrexate and dipyridamole in colorectal carcinoma. Cancer Treat Rep 71:821–824, 1987.
36. Higano C and Livingston R. Oral dipyridamole and methotrexate in human solid tumors: a toxicity trial. Cancer Chemother Pharmacol 23:259–262, 1989.
37. Woodcock TM, Gentile PS, Seeger J, Epremian BE, Hamm JT, Sheth SP, Sherrill EJ, Kellihan MJ, Lalley KA, and Allegra JC. A phase I study of dipyridamole and methotrexate (MTX). Proc Am Soc Clin Oncol 6:29, 1987.
38. Howell SB. Intraperitoneal chemotherapy in ovarian carcinoma. Contrib Oncol 29:72–83, 1988.
39. Goel R, Cleary SM, Horton C, Balis F, Zimm S, Kirmani S, and Howell SB. Selective intraperitoneal biochemical modulation of methotrexate by dipyridamole. J Clin Oncol 7:262–269, 1989.
40. Pinedo HM and Peters GFJ. Fluorouracil: biochemistry and pharmacology. J Clin Oncol 6:1653–1664, 1988.
41. Grem JL and Fischer PH. Augmentation of 5-fluorouracil cytotoxicity in human colon cancer cells by dipyridamole. Cancer Res 45:2967–2972, 1985.

42. Grem JL and Fischer PH. Alternation of fluorouracil metabolism in human colon cancer cells by dipyridamole with a selective increase in fluorodeoxyuridine monophosphate levels. Cancer Res 46:6191–6199, 1986.
43. Grem JL, Fischer PH, Mulcahy RT, Miller EM, Allegra CJ, and Fischer PH. Interaction of deoxyuridine with fluorouracil and dipyridamole in a human colon cancer cell line. Biochem Pharmacol 38:51–59, 1989.
44. Darnowski JW, Abate RA, and Handschumacher RE. Manipulation of tissue uridine pools with benzylacyclouridine and dipyridamole modifies fluorouracil therapy. Proc Am Assoc Cancer Res 29:474, 1988.
45. Lonn U, Lonn S, Nylen U, and Winblad G. 5-Fluoropyrimidine-induced DNA damage in human colon adenocarcinoma and its augmentation by the nucleoside transport inhibitor dipyridamole. Cancer Res 49:1085–1089, 1989.
46. Miller EM, Willson JKV, and Fischer PH. Folinic acid alters the mechanism by which dipyridamole (DP) increases the toxicity of fluorouracil (FUra) in human colon cancer cells. Proc Am Assoc Cancer Res 28:326, 1987.
47. Remick SC, Grem JL, Fischer PH, Tutsch KD, Alberti DB, Nieting LM, Tombes MB, Bruggink J, Willson JK, and Trump DL. Phase I trial of 5-fluorouracil and dipyridamole administered by seventy-two-hour concurrent continuous infusion. Cancer Res 50:2667–2772, 1990.
48. Budd JT, Jayaraj A, Grabowski A, Adelstein D, Baver L, Boyett J, Bukowski R, Murthy S, and Weick J. Phase I trial of dipyridamole with 5-fluorouracil and folinic acid. Cancer Res 50:7206–7211, 1990.
49. Schmoll H-J, Wilke H, Schober C, and Stahl M. High dose folinic acid (HDFA)/5-fluorouracil (FU)/dipyridamole (DP)—salvage after HDFA/FU-failure in colorectal cancer: a phase I study. Proc Am Soc Clin Oncol 7:114, 1988.
50. Allen S, Fine S, and Erlichman C. A phase II trial of 5-fluorouracil (5FU) and folinic acid (FA) plus dipyridamole (D) in patients with metastatic colorectal cancer (MCC). Proc Am Soc Clin Oncol 6:95, 1987.
51. Migeod F, Gerlach D, Kress M, Hoffman W, Farroukh R, and Seeber S. Sequentielle behandlung des progredient metastasierenden kolerektalen karzinoms mit 5-fluorouracil/folinsaure, dipyramidol und mitomycin C. Onkologie 11(Suppl. 2):14–20, 1988.
52. Buzaid AC, Alberts DS, Einspahr J, Mosley K, Peng YM, Tutsch K, Spears CP, and Garewal HS. Effect of dipyridamole on fluorodeoxyuridine in vitro and in cancer patients. Cancer Chemother Pharmacol 25:124–130, 1989.
53. Seeger J, Woodcock TM, Lalley KA, and Wieman TJ. Reduction of hepatotoxicity from intraarterial 2′,5 fluorodeoxyuridine (FUdR) by dipyridamole (DP). Proc Am Assoc Cancer Res 29:351, 1988.
54. Jamieson GP, Snook MB, Bradley TR, Bertoncello I, and Wiley JS. Transport and metabolism of 1-b-D-arabinofuranosylcytosine in human adenocarcinoma cells. Cancer Res 49:309–313, 1989.
55. King ME, Naporn A, Young B, and Howell SB. Modulation of cytarabine uptake and toxicity by dipyridamole. Cancer Treat Rep 68:361–363, 1984.
56. Kubota M, Takimoto T, Kitoh T, Tanizawa A, Kiriyama Y, Akiyama Y, and Mikawa H. Prevention of 1-β-D arabinofuranosylcytosine toxicity by 4-nitrobenzyl-6-thioinsine or dipyridamole in human leukemia cell lines. Anticancer Res 8:339–342, 1988.
57. Yang JL, White JC, and Capizzi RL. Enhanced retention of cytosine arabinoside and its metabolites and synergistic cytotoxicity by sequential treatment with dipyridamole in L5178Y leukemia. Cancer Chemother Pharmacol 26:135–138, 1990.
58. Chan TC. Augmentation of 1-beta-D-arabinofuranosylcytosine cytotoxicity in human tumor cells by inhibiting drug efflux. Cancer Res 49:2656–2660, 1989.
59. Earhart RH. Acivicin: a new antimetabolite. In: Concepts, Clinical Developments, and Therapeutic Advances in Cancer Chemotherapy, FM Muggia (ed). Martinus Nijhoff, Boston, 1987, pp. 161–181.
60. Zhen Y-S, Lui MS, and Weber G. Effects of acivicin and dipyridamole on hepatoma 3924A

cells. Cancer Res 43:1616–1619, 1983.
61. Fischer PH, Pamukcu R, Bittner G, and Willson JKV. Enhancement of the sensitivity of human colon cancer cells to growth inhibition by acivicin achieved through inhibition of nucleic acid precursor salvage by dipyridamole. Cancer Res 44:3355–3359, 1984.
62. Fischer PH, Willson JKV, Risueno C, Tutsch K, Bruggink J, Ranhosky A, and Trump DL. Biochemical assessment of the effects of acivicin and dipyridamole given as a continuous 72-hour infusion. Cancer Res 48:5591–5596, 1988.
63. Swyryd EA, Seaver SS, and Stark GR. N-(phosphonacetyl)-L-aspartate, a potent transition state analog inhibitor of aspartate transcarbamylase, blocks proliferation of mammalian cells in culture. J Biol Chem 249:6945–6950, 1974.
64. Levine RL, Hoogenraad NJ, and Kretchmer N. A review: biological and clinical aspects of pyrimidine metabolism. Pediatr Res 68:724–734, 1974.
65. Markman M, Chan TKC, Cleary S, and Howell SB. Phase I trial of combination therapy of cancer with N-phosphonacetyl-L-aspartic acid and dipyridamole. Cancer Chemother Pharmacol 19:80–83, 1987.
66. Chan TCK, Young B, King ME, Taetle R, and Howell SB. Modulation of the activity of PALA by dipyridamole. Cancer Treat Rep 69:425–530, 1985.
67. Chan TCK and Howell SB. Mechanism of synergy between N-phosphonacetyl-L-asparate and dipyridamole in a human ovarian carcinoma cell line. Cancer Res 45:3598–3564, 1985.
68. Chan TCK, Markman M, Cleary S, and Howell SB. Plasma uridine changes in cancer patients treated with the combination of dipyridamole and N-phosphoacetyl-L-aspartate. Cancer Res 46:3168–3172, 1986.
69. Howell SB, Vick J, Andrews PA, Velury S, and Sanga R. Biochemical modulation of cisplatin. In: Platinum and Other Metal Coordination Compounds in Cancer Chemotherapy, M Nicolini (ed). Martinus Nijhoff, Boston, 1987.
70. Howell SB, Hom DK, Sanga R, Vick JS, and Chan TCK. Dipyridamole enhancement of etoposide sensitivity. Cancer Res 49:4147–4153, 1989.
71. Howell SB, Hom D, Sanga R, Vick JS, and Abramson IS. Comparison of the synergistic potentiation of etoposide, doxorubicin, and vinblastine cytotoxicity by dipyridamole. Cancer Res 49:3178–3183, 1989.
72. Hirose M, Takeda E, Ninomiya T, Kuroda Y, and Miyao M. Synergistic inhibitory effects of dipyridamole and vincristine on the growth of human leukaemia and lyphoma cell lines. Br J Cancer 56:413–417, 1987.
73. Kusumoto H, Maechara Y, Anai H, Kusumoto T, and Sugimachi K. Potentiation of adriamycin cytotoxicity by dipyridamole against HeLa cells in vitro and Sarcoma 180 cells in vivo. Cancer Res 48:1208–1212, 1988.
74. Yin MB, Bankusli I, Frank C, and Rustum YM. Modulation of doxorubicin-induced DNA lesions by verapamil, DMDP and dipyridamole in resistant P388 cell lines. Anticancer Res 10:327–332, 1990.
75. Newell DR, O'Connor PM, Bishop J, Calvert AH, and Harrap KR. Dipyridamole induced inhibition of thymidine incorporation in vivo and potentiation of CB3717 cytotoxicity in vitro. Br J Cancer 52:431, 1985.
76. Curtin NJ, Harris AL, and Aherne GW. Mechanism of cell death following thymidylate. Synthase inhibition: 2′-deoxyuridine-5′-triphosphate accumulation, DNA damage, and growth inhibition following exposure to CB3717 and dipyridamole. Cancer Res 51:2346–2352, 1991.
77. Kung G-J and Kimball AP. Dipyridamole enhancement of toxicity to L1210 cells by deoxyadenosine and deoxycoformycin combinations in vitro. Cancer Res 44:461–466, 1984.
78. Janowska-Wieczorek A and Cass CE. Protection of human hematopoietic stem cells from tubericidin toxicity by inhibitors of nucleoside transport. Proc Am Assoc Cancer Res 28:409, 1987.
79. Cordon-Cardo C, O'Brien JP, Casals D, Rittman-Grauer L, Biedler JL, Melamed MR, and Bertino JR. Multidrug-resistance gene (P-glycoprotein) is expressed by endothelial cells at blood-brain barrier sites. Proc Natl Acad Sci USA 86:695–698, 1989.

3. Pharmacology and clinical investigation of SR-2508 (etanidazole)

Peter J. O'Dwyer and Frank P. LaCreta

Introduction

The common, slow-growing solid tumors remain refractory to current chemotherapeutic strategies. Resistance appears, in part, to be a consequence of the abnormal metabolic environment of solid tumors. It is proposed that the disordered vascular development in the growing tumor mass results in a proportion of cells being remote from capillaries; the increased diffusion distance leads to hypoxia, low glucose concentrations, and reduced cellular pH [reviewed in 1]. Cells in this hypoxic environment pose a particular problem, because while quiescent under hypoxic conditions, they may be recruited into the proliferative fraction as a tumor shrinks in response to therapy. Tumor regrowth during reoxygenation following radiation therapy illustrates this phenomenon. It has long been recognized that in their quiescent state, hypoxic cells are resistant both to radiation and to electrophilic cytotoxic drug [2, 3]. The proportion of hypoxic cells in a tumor is in part a function of tumor size; but even small tumors (1 mm in diameter) may have hypoxic fractions ranging from 10 to 30% [4]. The tumor types in which significant hypoxic fractions have been identified include all the common solid tumors, especially lung, colon, head and neck, and breast cancers [5].

The basis for hypoxic cell resistance to alkylating agents is not well established and is probably multifactorial, including a) poor penetration of blood-borne drug to remote tumor cells; b) protection of quiescent (non-cycling) cells from cell-cycle-specific agents; c) enhanced conjugation of drugs to glutathione and other intracellular thiols; and d) altered drug metabolism in a hypoxic environment. Several of these mechanisms overlap with those more usually associated with acquired drug resistance, and some studies indicate that these processes may be common responses to a variety of stimuli [6]. For example, gene amplification (of the DHFR gene) may occur in response to a brief hypoxic exposure [7, 8]; cell culture under hypoxic conditions has been associated with an increase in the specific activity of glutathione-S-transferase (GST); and resistant cells with both elevated GST levels and the MDR phenotype have been described [9].

Franco M. Muggia (ed.), NEW DRUGS, CONCEPTS AND RESULTS IN CANCER CHEMOTHERAPY.

Kluwer Academic Publishers, Boston. *ISBN 0-7923-1253-8*

Therefore, glutathione and its associated enzymes, currently targets for strategies to reverse acquired resistance, may also be important in the phenomenon of hypoxic cell resistance.

Two approaches to increasing the sensitivity of hypoxic cells to cytoxic drugs are currently under active investigation: a) the development of drugs that are selectively activated in the reducing environment of the hypoxic cell, such as mitomycin C [10], and b) the use of 'oxygen-mimetic' compounds capable of diffusing into hypoxic cells. Several analogs of mitomycin are under development in the United States and Japan, while other drug classes activated by bioreduction are in advanced preclinical studies, especially nitroimidazole-alkylating agent conjugates and benzotriazine-di-N-oxides. Indeed *increasing* tumor hypoxia (with vasodilators such as hydralazine, which result in a steal phenomenon) potentiates bioreductively activated drugs in a variety of in vivo systems [11].

Of the O_2-mimetic drugs, 2-nitroimidazoles are the best studied and are the focus of this review. A series of these drugs has been evaluated in clinical and preclinical studies in the last 8 years (figure 1). These electrophilic drugs restore the sensitivity of hypoxic cells to radiation in vitro and in vivo [12]. The prototype, misonidazole (MISO), has been evaluated extensively in the clinic. Though MISO exhibited dose-modifying factors (DMF) of 1.8–2.4, depending on the experimental conditions, large-scale randomized studies failed to show any benefit from its use with radiation therapy [13, 14]. The dose-limiting neurotoxicity was shown to relate principally to the lipophilicity of MISO, which favored CNS penetration [15].

Desmethylmisonidiazole, a metabolite of misonidazole that retains sensitizing activity, and is slightly less lipophilic, was also evaluated clinically: no toxicity advantage over MISO was demonstrated and the compound was dropped. Benznidazole (an antihelminthic) and Ro 03-8799 have been evaluated in clinical trials in Europe [16, 17]. In the United States, the major sensitizer selected for clinical development is SR-2508 (recently given the generic name *etanidazole*), a compound with an octanol-water partition coeffient of 0.046 versus 0.45 for misonidazole and an equally potent radiosensitizer [18]. SR2508 has begun phase I testing as a radiosensitizer; these studies have shown that cumulative doses three- to fourfold higher than those of misonidazole are well tolerated [19]; SR-2508 is now in randomized trials to assess its role as a radiosensitizer.

Nitroimidazoles as chemosensitizers

In addition to sensitizing hypoxic cells to radiation, the nitroimidazoles restore the sensitivity of hypoxic cells to cytotoxic drugs. This effect was first demonstrated by Clement et al. and Rose et al. [20, 21], and is particularly marked for alkylating agents [22]. Misonidazole enhanced the antitumor activity of cyclophosphamide in the M5076 tumor and Lewis lung [20]. In

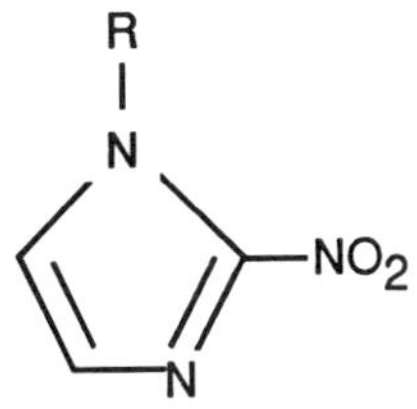

2-Nitroimidazoles

R	
$CH_2CH(OH)CH_2OCH_3$	Misonidazole
$CH_2CH(OH)CH_2OH$	Desmethyl misonidazole
$CH_2CONHCH_2$ – Phenyl	Benznidazole
$CH_2CONHCH_2CH_2OH$	SR-2508
$CH_2CON(CH_2CH_2OH)_2$	SR-2555
$CH_2CH(OH)CH_2OCH_2$ – Piperidine	Ro 03 - 8799

Figure 1. Structure of some 2-nitroimidazoles of clinical interest.

M5076, the nitroimidazole also potentiated the activity of L-phenylalanine mustard, a nitrosurea, and aziridinylbenzoquinone, but not that of cisplatin. The antitumor activity of L-phenylalanine mustard and cyclophosphamide were potentiated by factors of 2.2 and 1.8, respectively, while myelotoxicity was increased only by 1.2- and 1.3-fold. At equimolar doses, SR2508 enhances the activity of CTX and L-PAM as effectively as MISO [23, 24]. Projections based on the higher plasma levels that may be achieved with SR-2508 suggest that SR-2508 will achieve superior sensitizing effects in the clinic [24]. Further, the in vivo study of Clement and colleagues, and numerous in vitro studies (figure 2), show that maximum sensitizing efficacy increases both with the dose of cyclophosphamide and that of the nitroimidazole. Since there is no evident plateau on these curves, it is clearly rational to attempt to give the highest dose possible of SR2508 for chemosensitization.

It is probable that the mechanistic basis for radiosensitizing and chemosensitizing effects are different: The former is dependent on high drug concentrations at the time of irradiation and is fully expressed immediately when the drug is added to the system. Chemosensitization, on the other hand, in enhanced by preincubation of cells with the sensitizing drug, and the phenomenon persists following drug removal [25]. This suggests that chemosensitization may depend upon either metabolism of SR2508 to 'active' species (by a series of one-electron reductions in hypoxic cells) and/or the interaction of such species with macromolecular targets such as DNA [26]. The potential mechanisms described to date are detailed (table 1).

Finally, it should be noted that nitroimidazoles are cytotoxic to cells, but only under conditions of hypoxia [26]. The basis for this is not understood, though drug treatment-associated DNA strand breaks have been described, and binding of labeled SR2508 to DNA is reported. Direct cytotoxicity of nitroimidazoles to hypoxic cells, which occurs at concentrations higher than

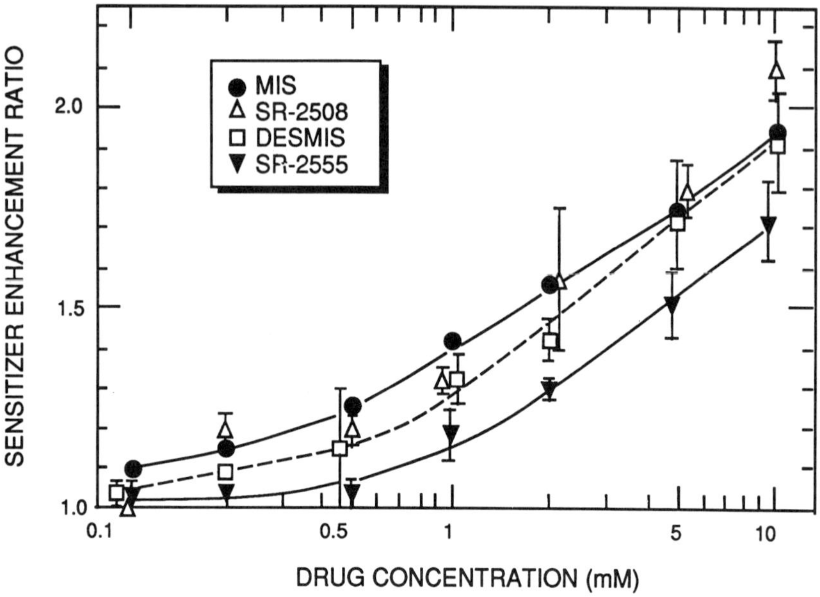

Figure 2. Sensitizer enhancement ratios as a function of nitroimidazole concentration in CHO HA-1 cells in vitro. (From Brown et al., Int J Radiat Oncol Biol Phys 7:695, 1981. With permission.)

Table 1. Possible mechanisms of chemosensitization of alkylating agent action by 2-nitroimidazoles

1. Altered alkylator pharmacokinetics
2. Increased DNA strand breaks/cross-links
3. Inhibition of DNA repair
4. Depletion of glutathione
5. Inhibition of glutathione-dependent detoxifying enzymes

those required for sensitization, is not considered to be a likely mechanism for their sensitizing effects.

Cellular metabolism of nitroimidazoles

Nitroimidazoles express neither their cytotoxic nor their sensitizing properties under aerobic conditions. Under oxic conditions, metabolism of the side chain may occur to a variable extent [18], and redox cycling at the 2-NO_2 group has been described [27] under hypoxia; however, the 2-nitro group is subject to successive 1-electron reduction steps, ending with the amine, R-NH_2 [27].

$$R\text{-}NO_2 \rightarrow R\text{-}NO_2 \rightarrow R\text{-}NO \rightarrow R\text{-}NHOH \rightarrow R\text{-}NH_2$$

At each step, a free radical may be formed; however, few of these radicals are likely to have significant stability in vivo. The initial anion radical may be produced in vitro by numerous enzymes, including NADPH-dependent cytochrome c reductase, cytochrome P450 reductase(s), xanthine oxidase, and aldehyde oxidase [26, 28]. The importance of each of these enzymes in mediating the 'nitroreductase' effect may vary from one tissue to another; several exist in isozymic forms, and varying affinity for substrate may account for differences in nitroanion formation [28]. Further sequential reduction of the anion radical occurs in hypoxic cells, resulting in the nitroso, hydroxylamine, and amine derivatives. Free radicals generated in these reactions may themselves react with macromolecules, a plausible mechanism of both cytotoxicity and sensitization. Alternatively, they may react with oxygen to yield superoxide and subsequently hydroxyl radical through a Fenton-like reaction. In normally oxic cells, reductive metabolism beyond the nitroradical anion does not appear to occur; the electron is transferred to O_2 to form a superoxide radical that is dismutated with the production of H_2O_2. This regenerates the parent compound, which becomes susceptible to reduction again. The continuous production of superoxide by redox cycling may occur in oxic cells [27], however, reduction to the nitroso intermediate or beyond appears to be required for cytotoxicity [29].

Wong and Agrawal have shown that both misonidazole and SR2508 are reduced by preparations of liver cytosol and liver microsomal fractions under hypoxic conditions [30]. A similar effect may be obtained with purified xanthine oxidase; each system requires the addition of exogenous NADPH. These investigators also demonstrated that depletion of glutathione from the hepatic subcellular fractions diminished their capacity to reduce nitroimidazoles. The effects of nitroreduction on glutathione metabolizing enzymes (such as GSTs) have not been studied. It is likely that the active intermediates that result from nitroreduction produce more profound changes in GSH levels in hypoxic than in oxic cells.

Cellular effects of the nitroimidazoles

The several cellular effects of the nitroimidazoles are dependent upon their metabolism. In oxic cells, the unpaired electron of the radical anion is rapidly shunted to H_2O_2; in hypoxic cells, persistence of the free radical is associated with depletion of glutathione [25], probably through the formation of GSH-nitroimidazole conjugates [31]. In vitro studies have also described inhibition of GST at clinically achievable levels of the sensitizer [32].

The role of GSH depletion in the sensitization phenomenon was investigated by Taylor et al. [33]. They showed that cells depleted of GSH by diethylmaleate are further sensitized to LPAM by MISO exposure. Treat-

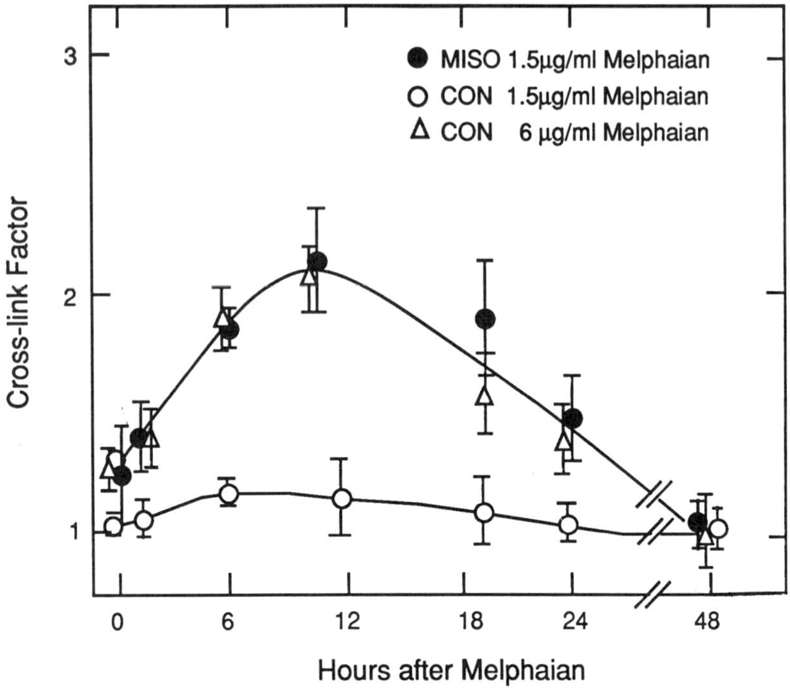

Figure 3. Removal of L-PAM cross-links in control and misonidazole-pretreated Chinese hamster ovary cells. (From Taylor et al., Cancer Res 43:3175, 1983. With permission.)

ment with MISO plus LPAM results in an increase in the number of interstrand cross-links over those detectable with LPAM alone; the curve for MISO/LPAM 1.5 µg/ml is superimposable upon LPAM 6 µg/ml, implying a fourfold sensitizer enhancement ratio (figure 3). However, there was no effect on the kinetics of cross-link formation or repair. These data indicate that MISO may inhibit the cell's ability to detoxify LPAM. Alternatively, the additional sensitization achieved in GSH-depleted cells may be a result of GST inhibition or the direct action of the sensitizer upon DNA.

While an effect at the cellular level is considered most likely, nitroimidazoles have been reported to retard the plasma elimination of alkylating agents [34]. The resulting increase in the plasma area under the concentration-time curve (AUC) has been proposed to contribute to the apparent interaction of nitroimidazoles and alkylators in rodents and humans [34]. In a phase I study, Tutsch et al. showed that SR-2508 had no effect on the pharmacokinetics of cyclophosphamide [35]. A definitive answer will require a similar assessment of the kinetics of the active alkylating species derived from cyclophosphamide. In another phase I study, we have found that cyclophosphamide has no influence on SR 2508 pharmacokinetics [36].

Further investigation of the cellular pharmacology of SR2508 and of the mechanism of chemosensitization will be important to determine how best to use SR2508 in treatment regimens. A fuller description of the interaction of SR2508 with GSH and GST will, in turn, indicate how the biochemical environment of hypoxic cells may be altered to restore or increase sensitivity to cytotoxic drugs.

Preclinical pharmacology of the nitroimidazoles

Analytical Methods

In general nitroimidazoles are readily measured in a variety of body fluids and tissues. The available methodology has been summarized in detail by Workman [18]. While ultraviolet spectrophotometry (300–350 nm), thin-layer chromatography, and paper chromatography have been described for nitroimidazole assay, high-pressure liquid chromatography (HPLC) is preferred. While the description of the following analytical method is specific for etanidazole, it should be noted that similar HPLC techniques have been described for various other nitroimidazoles [15].

Etanidazole concentrations in various types of biological samples are readily determined using HPLC with ultraviolet absorbance detection. The technique employed in our laboratory involves deproteinization of plasma and urine samples with methanol, followed by centrifugation to remove all insoluble material. Tissue samples are processed in a similar manner; the tissue is weighed, homogenized in methanol, and centrifuged. The methanbolic supernatant is removed and evaporated to dryness under a stream of nitrogen, and the resulting extract is dissolved in mobile phase for analysis. The reverse-phase HPLC system utilizes a octadecylsilyl column (we use a 300 × 4 mm C18 μBondapak analytical column) with a mobile phase consisting of 5% methanol in water. The flow rate is 2 ml/min and detection is by ultraviolet absorbance at 320 nm. By utilizing the unusual absorbance maximum of this compound, interference by endogenous substances is virtually eliminated. The chromatographic procedure requires 6 minutes per run, with etanidazole eluting at 3.6 minutes. No other nitro-containing species have been detected in plasma, urine, or tissue samples using this analytical procedure, which supports the observations of others demonstrating the lack of metabolism of the hydrophilic side chain [37]. The precision of this technique is evident in the day-to-day coefficient of variation (CV) of 5–10% from 0.1 to 50 μg/ml, and the within-day CV of less than 4%. The lower limit of quantitation is 50 ng/ml, and the detector response is linear up to 50 μg/ml.

While determination of the parent compound is relatively easy, quantitation of the reduction products of etanidazole is much more difficult. Various techniques have been applied to measure the reduction products of other nitroimidazoles. Flockhart et al. [38] have demonstrated the amine product of MISO in urine using precolumn derivatization with 2,4-dinitrofluorobenzene followed by normal-phase HPLC. Likewise, normal-phase HPLC has been used to illustrate the hydroxylamine product [39]. Promising techniques to study the reductive metabolism of nitroimidazoles include gas-liquid chromatography-mass spectrometry and electron paramagnetic resonance (EPR). Koch et al. [40] have studied the ring-cleaved products of MISO and metronidazole using the former technique. Rao and Mason [41] have used EPR to detect radicals resulting from the sequential one-electron reduction products of nitroimidazoles. Chemical evidence of radical formation in the radiochemical reduction of nitroimidazoles has been obtained in the studies of Rauth et al. [42]. The application of some of these methodologies to in vivo studies may help to clarify the importance of metabolism in the sensitizing action of nitroimidazoles.

Preclinical pharmacokinetics

All the clinically used nitroimidazoles have been studied in rodents and/or dogs. The data concerning misonidazole and other analogues have been summarized in some detail [18] and will not be considered further here. Lipophilic nitroimidazoles, such as MISO, are cleared principally by metabolism, while hydrophilic analogues (e.g., SR2508) are cleared by renal excretion.

SR2508 pharmacokinetics in mice are independent of dose [37]. Following IV administration, plasma elimination is biphasic, with a terminal half-life of approximately 1 hour. Total body clearance of SR2508 is approximately twice as rapid as that of misonidazole. Elimination is primarily renal, and 89% of an administrated dose is found unchanged in the urine. Induction of microsomal enzymes with phenobarbital had no effect on SR2508 clearance.

In the dog the half-life is longer, varying from 2 to 3 hours [43]. Total body clearance is 0.21 l/kg/hr. As with the mouse, renal excretion predominates (89%). The oral bioavailability of SR2508 was also studied in the dog; 86% of an administered dose was absorbed (compared to 92% for misonidazole). However, absorption was slow and peak plasma levels were less than one fifth of those resulting from IV administration. As noted by Workman [44], these preclinical models were reliable in predicting the human pharmacology of SR 2508.

Intratumoral SR 2508

The systemic administration of radiosensitizers has been limited by the appearance of dose-limiting toxicity at suboptimal sensitizer levels [45, 46]. This finding has led to the evaluation of alternative routes of drug delivery to the hypoxic fraction of the tumor: a route that is currently being investigated is direct intratumoral administration of the drug. Recent laboratory studies suggest that intratumoral injection of radiosensitizers may be more effective than systemic administration [47, 48]. At Fox Chase, injection of a supersaturated solution of etanidazole into the tumor, followed by radiotherapy, resulted in a significantly smaller ($p < .05$) tumor volume 9 days post-treatment, compared to a group given the sensitizer by the intraperitoneal (IP) route [49]. In a later study, the corresponding tumor and plasma concentrations were measured spectrophotometrically [50]. The intratumorally injected group had tumor levels 20 times higher and plasma levels 0.2 times as high as the group receiving the same dose of etanidazole by IP administration. Using these data, a DMF of 1.88 was calculated for intratumoral etanidazole, which was significantly different from that obtained following IP dosing (DMF-1.28).

To further investigate the utility of this route of administration, we investigated the pharmacokinetics and tissue distribution of etanidazole in cats bearing spontaneously occurring oral squamous cell carcinoma (SCC). Feline SCC is the most common oropharyngeal neoplasm in the cat and shares many similarities with human head and neck cancer. The pharmacokinetics of etanidazole were determined following separate IV and intratumoral administration to the same animal [51]. This design allowed each animal to serve as its own control and permitted calculation of systemic availability. Pharmacokinetic studies were performed in four cats; plasma and urine drug concentrations were measured by HPLC. Following IV infusion the plasma elimination of etanidazole was biexponential ($\alpha t_{1/2}$ = 17.8 minutes; $\beta t_{1/2}$ = 3.2 hours). The volume of the central compartment was 0.28 l/kg and the steady-state volume of distribution was 0.60 l/kg, indicating distribution into extracellular fluid and total body water, respectively, in agreement with that found in various species, including humans. Following intratumoral administration, the systemic availability of etanidazole was 61%. Tumor drug levels in one cat during treatment showed a tumor to plasma concentration ratio at the time of radiotherapy (30 minutes postinjection) almost five times higher following intratumoral compared to IV administration. These results suggest that the intratumoral route may enhance the therapeutic index of nitroimidazoles and warrants further investigation.

Pharmacology of nitroimidazoles in humans

Pharmacokinetics

In phase I trial, we measured concentrations of etanidazole in plasma and urine after intravenous dosing (table 2) [36]. Following a 30-minute constant-rate infusion, the plasma disappearance curve of etanidazole fit a two-compartment open model with a distribution half-life of 20 minutes, followed by a terminal elimination phase with a half-life ranging from 4 to 6 hours.

Table 2. Pharmacokinetics of etanidazole in humans following IV administration

Dose	1 g/m^2	2.5 g/m^2	3.25 g/m^2	4.2 g/m^2	5.5 g/m^2	7.2 g/m^2
Plasma						
$t_{1/2\alpha}$, hr	0.48	0.30	0.49	0.39	0.31	0.35
$t_{1/2\beta}$, hr	5.4	5.1	5.1	5.4	5.8	5.3
AUC, μg/hr/ml	281	786	878	833	2047	2214
Volumes						
V_c, l/m^2	10.96	7.65	9.47	11.85	7.2	8.3
Vd_{ss}, l/m^2	24.5	21.4	22.2	32.3	20.0	21.4
Clearance						
Cl, total ml/min/m^2	65.7	61.3	64.2	94.0	46.6	56.6
Cl renal, ml/min/m^2	43.2	45.8	48.1	61.7	36.9	42.1
Cl%	65.7	74.6	75.0	65.7	79.3	74.4

The area under the plasma concentration versus time curve increased proportionally with dose (from 1 to 15.2 g/m^2), indicating that the pharmacokinetics were not dose dependent over this range. From the estimated volumes of distribution, we concluded that the volume of the central compartment approximated that of extracellular water, and the steady-state volume of distribution was equivalent to the volume of total body water. These data indicate that etanidazole readily enters cells and agree with preclinical studies of etanidazole distribution [43]. Etanidazole elimination occurs primarily through renal mechanisms. Renal clearance is 50–100 ml/min, which is close to GFR, and accounts for 70% of total body clearance. The extent to which metabolism and biliary excretion contributes to etanidazole elimination is unknown at the present time.

Similar results were obtained in the trial of Tutsch et al. [35]: a biphasic plasma elimination curve with terminal half-life of 5.9 hours, total body clearance of 55 ml/min/m^2, and apparent volume of distribution at steady state of 23.1 l/m^2. In addition, these authors showed no alteration of pharmacokinetic parameters with repeat dosing.

Pharmacodynamic effects of SR2508 in humans

SR2508 at doses as low as 1 g/m^2 was found to inhibit GST activity in peripheral mononuclear cells (PMNs) by over 50%. The activity in red blood cells was unaffected. Depletion of PMN GSH levels parallels the inhibition of GST. At higher doses more complete inhibition of GST and profound depletion of GSH pools is noted (figure 4). However, considerable interpatient variability in these biochemical effects was noted. These differences cannot be explained on the basis of plasma pharmacokinetics, which exhibited little interpatient variability. They may related to either interindividual differences in SR2508 activation or to phenotypic differences in GST isoenzyme expression. Preliminary data have also been obtained from

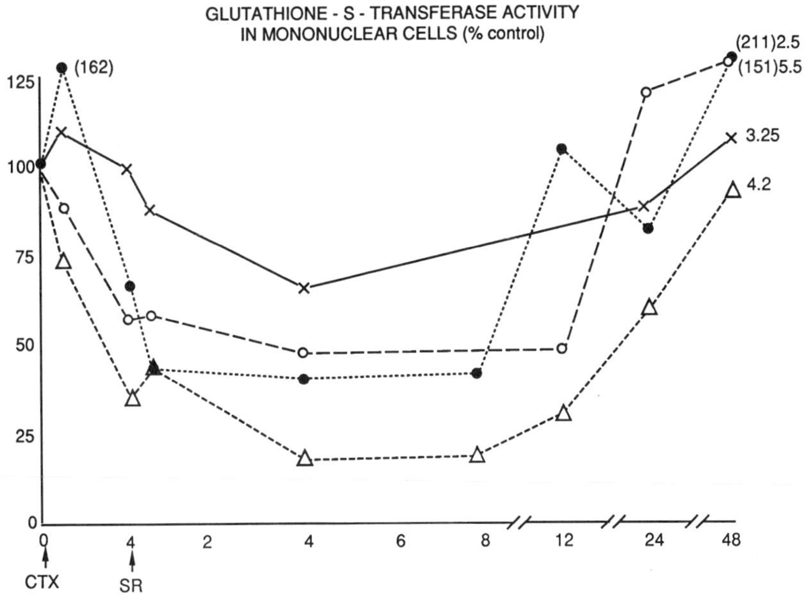

Figure 4. Glutathione S-transferase activity in peripheral mononuclear cells of patients treated with cyclophosphamide and escalating doses of etanidazole (2.5–5.5 g/m^2).

biopsies performed in three patients following SR2508 treatment. These limited data show results that are concordant with the PMN data in that transferase inhibition and GSH depletion is observed at the 12-hour point. Determination of the kinetics of recovery of enzyme activity will require larger numbers of patients to elucidate the optimal schedule of drug administration for future phase II studies.

Clinical studies with SR 2508

Phase I studies of SR 2508 as a radiosensitizer

The initial phase I studies of SR2508 were performed by Coleman and colleagues in the Radiation Therapy Oncology Group (RTOG) [19, 52]. Intravenous bolus doses from 1.3 to 3.7 g/m^2 were tolerated without acute toxicity. Two schedules were evaluated: three times weekly dosing for 3–5 weeks and daily dosing with the use of a 'split course' (i.e., 2 weeks of SR2508 treatment with radiation therapy, 2 weeks of radiation therapy alone, followed by a final 2 weeks of both modalities). An exploration of the maximum tolerated single dose was not pursued in these studies. A dose of 2 g/m^2 was calculated to produce a tumor concentration of approximately 100 μg/ml, which would theoretically yield a sensitizer enhancement ratio of 1.5–1.7.

Of greater concern than the single dose in the radiation therapy studies was the maximum tolerated cumulative dose. As with previously studied nitroimidazoles, a peripheral sensory neuropathy became dose limiting after repeated drug administration. The cumulative total dose at which the peripheral neuropathy occurred was markedly variable between patients and had an onset at cumulative doses from 21.6 g/m^2 to over 40 g/m^2. On the more frequent schedules of administration, there was a clear trend for patients to tolerate higher cumulative drug doses. Coleman and colleagues also noted a relationship between the total area under the curve in a given patient (extrapolated from a single measured AUC multiplied by the number of drug doses administered) and the risk of neurotoxicity [53]. In the model used, the predictive value of the pharmacokinetic criterion was considerably better than that of the total dose administered. Validation of this model is being attempted in a group-wide study.

Based on these phase I studies, SR2508 is now in phase II and phase III clinical trials as a radiosensitizer. The key trials are being conducted in head and neck cancer, bladder cancer, and cervical cancer. SR2508 is used in combination with curative radiation therapy at 2 g/m^2 three times weekly to a total dose of 34 g/m^2. Preliminary toxicity data from these studies indicate that this regimen is well tolerated in an expanded patient population.

SR 2508 is also being studied in combination with Ro 03-8799, a basic lipophilic nitroimidazole that does not cause peripheral neuropathy. The dose of Ro 03-8799 is limited to 0.75–1.0 g/m^2 by an acute transient central nervous system syndrome [54]. Preclinical data indicate that the combined use of SR 2508 and Ro 03-8799 may yield additive radiosensitization [44]. A phase I trial of the combination was initiated on the basis non-overlapping toxicity: results show that Ro 03-8799 appears to limit the total dose of SR 2508 to 24–28 g/m^2 [17, 55]. This suggests that Ro 03-8799 may potentiate the neurotoxicity of SR 2508. However, at these doses a DMF of 1.5 may be expected from the combination [56].

Phase I trials of SR2508 as a chemosensitizer

The major issue in designing an initial regimen of SR2508 in combination with cyclophosphamide (CTX) was the schedule of drug administration. Preclinical in vivo studies had produced conflicting results concerning the necessity for preincubation. Siemann and Mulcahy showed that the optimal schedule appeared to be when the alkylating agent (CCNU, melphalan) and the sensitizer (misonidazole, SR 2508) were given close to the same time, even though in some tumors the role of preincubation with a sensitizer was more effective [25]. On the other hand, Clement et al. showed that in the M5076 murine model, a twofold increase in activity resulted when the miso and CTX were administered close to simultaneously. In the study conducted at Fox Chase Cancer Center, we elected to schedule the maximum plasma alkylating activity and maximum sensitizer levels at approximately the same time, and to perform biochemical measurements that could guide us to future schedule selection. Since cyclophosphamide has no alkylating activity until metabolized to its 4-hydroxy derivative (levels of which peak at 4 hours), administration of CTX preceded that of SR2508 by a 4-hour interval. The design of the study is shown in table 3. SR2508, as a single agent given 1 week prior to the combined administration of CTX SR2508, permits an assessment of

1. Dose dependency of SR2508 pharmacokinetics, and
2. Influence of CTX on SR2508 pharmacokinetics

Tutsch and colleagues evaluated the opposite schedule of administration. In their study, SR2508 administration preceded that of CTX by 2 hours [35].

The dose of SR2508 has now been escalated in combination with cyclophosphamide from 2.5 to 15 g/m^2. At the 7.2 g/m^2, dose-limiting myelosuppression required a 25% reduction in CTX dose (table 4). This dose reduction was undertaken to allow a definitive determination of the MTD of SR 2508 on this schedule, for future integration into dose intense regimens.

The major side effect of cyclophosphamide when administered alone is myelosuppression, affecting principally white blood cells. This is not a known side effect of SR2508, though it appears to increase in severity in proportion to the dose of SR2508 (table 5). This observation may have several explanations:

Table 3. Design of phase I study of cyclophosphamide and etanidazole

Level	Course #1	Course #2 and subsequent	# Patients
1	SR2508 1 g/m^2	CTX 1 g/m^2 4h → SR2508 2.5 g/m^2	6
2	SR2508 1 g/m^2	CTX 1 g/m^2 → SR2508 3.25 g/m^2	6
3	SR2508 1 g/m^2	CTX 1 g/m^2 → SR2508 4.2 g/m^2	6
4	SR2508 1 g/m^2	CTX 1 g/m^2 → SR2508 5.6 g/m^2	6
5	SR2508 1 g/m^2	CTX 1 g/m^2 → SR2508 7.5 g/m^2	6
		Continue 33% increments	

Table 4. Phase I study of etanidazole and cyclophosphamide: Dose levels tested

Level	Week 1 SR2508 Dose	Week 2 CTX Dose	Week 2 SR2508 Dose	#Pts
1	1	1000	2.5	6
2	1	1000	3.25	6
3	1	1000	4.2	6
4	1	1000	5.5	6
5	1	1000	7.2	4
6	7.2	1000	7.2	3
7	9.4	750	9.4	6
8	12.2	750	12.2	5
9	15	750	15	3

Table 5. Myelosuppression following administration of escalating doses of etanidazole in combination with cyclophosphamide (750 or 1000 mg/m^2)

Dose (g/m^2)	No.	WBC Toxicity—Grade				
		0	1	2	3	4
2.5	6	0	3	1	1	1
3.25	6	1	1	1	2	0
4.2	6	0	1	2	1	2
5.5	6	1	1	0	2	2
7.2	7	0	0	1	5	1
9.4	6	2	1	0	3	0
12.2	5	2	0	2	0	1
15	3	1	0	1	0	1

1. SR2508 at these doses may itself by myelosuppressive.
2. SR2508 at these doses may alter the plasma pharmacokinetics and/or the metabolism of cyclophosphamide.
3. SR2508 may influence the effects of cyclophosphamide at a cellular level by inhibiting its detoxification or by delaying the repair of the DNA lesion. It has recently demonstrated that GSH is directly involved in DNA repair, and the interaction of SR2508 and GSH is being studied further.

The other major clinical toxicity attributable to SR2508 is neurotoxicity. Based on previous work with misonidazole, it was anticipated that central neurotoxicity (confusion, hallucinations, etc.) might become a problem at the higher doses. Peripheral neurotoxicity in the form of sensorimotor neuropathy was projected to limit the total dose of SR2508 and to reflect the cumulative toxicity of the drug. However, we found no evidence of central neurotoxicity at any dose studied on this trial. At doses higher than 7.2 g/m^2, we evaluated the patients before and at various times after SR2508 administration using the 'mini-mental' test, as developed by investigators in the Department of Neurology at Johns Hopkins. Patients' scores did not change following treatment. At doses $\geqslant$9.36 g/m^2, however, a syndrome of acute peripheral neuropathy consisting of pain radiating down the extremities from the hip or shoulder girdles, and having onset from 4 to 12 hours after treatment, began to appear. The severity of this syndrome was dose related and has turned out to be dose limiting at 15.2 g/m^2. At this dose, two patients required high doses of morphine to relieve the acute pain. Resolution of symptoms occurs within 12–18 hours, and curiously, symptoms are never as severe on second and subsequent courses of treatment.

Cumulative toxicity is difficult to analyze in a phase I study, since the average number of courses administered is generally low. RTOG investigators had shown that a total dose of SR2508 of 21–40.8 g/m^2 was maximally tolerable in their studies [19]. A fuller picture of results on this schedule will emerge as patients at the two highest levels are treated for longer periods of time, but already there is an indication that the maximum tolerated *cumulative* dose may be in excess of 37 g/m^2, since two patients tolerated a total of 60 g/m^2. One of the two developed a peripheral neuropathy, which is resolving.

Clinical-pharmacokinetic correlations

While analysis is incomplete, the pharmacokinetics of SR2508 correlate closely with a number of patient characteristics. Consistent with the importance of renal elimination, total body clearance of SR2508 and creatinine clearance are highly correlated ($p = .0001$), as are AUC and Cl_r ($p = .001$). Cl_{TB} is also significantly related to WBC and neutrophil toxicity ($p < .01$). Since this correlation is better than that for either AUC or SR2508 dose, it would appear that the clearance of SR2508 and that of active metabolites of cyclophosphamide may be related.

Future studies

The phase I studies at Fox Chase and Wisconsin are in close accord concerning the definition of the MTD of SR2508. The optimal schedule of SR2508/cyclophosphamide administration is suggested from the biochemical findings in both peripheral mononuclear cells and tumor biopsy specimens. The effect of SR2508 on glutathione and related enzymes requires 8–12 hours to become manifest. We have recently demonstrated a similar time course in tumors and normal tissues of mice (PJ O'Dwyer, unpublished data). Accordingly, the optimal schedule would probably administer SR2508 4–8 hours before cyclophosphamide administration. Selection of the optimal dose should take into account the following:

1. Dose-related increases in GSH depletion were not observed beyond 5.5 g/m^2.
2. At SR2508 7.2 g/m^2, a dose reduction of CTX was required.
3. While the maximum cumulative dose of SR2508 seems higher with this schedule of administration, it is likely to lie in the range of 40–60 g/m^2.
4. It seems desirable to select a schedule that will permit administration of SR2508 with every dose of alkylating agent for a minimum of six to eight courses. For this reason a suitable phase II dose would be 6–8 g/m^2. At Fox Chase, we will soon pilot this dose on the schedule described, in preparation for phase II and phase III studies.

Having established a biochemically rational dose and schedule of SR2508 on clinical and pharmacologic grounds, the further development of this regimen requires careful consideration. The potential for reversing hypoxic cell resistance to alkylating agents with nitroimidazoles will be explored in one, or at most two, large randomized studies. Therefore, it seems appropriate to choose carefully the tumors to be studied and the regimens in which SR2508 should be incorporated. In selecting a disease to be treated, the following principles seem sensible:

1. Cyclophosphamide should be 'standard therapy,' either alone or in combination.
2. The tumor should be known to have a significant fraction of hypoxic cells.
3. A combination of the 'best regimens' for this disease with SR2508 should be feasible on grounds of toxicity.
4. The tumor should be relatively common, so that sufficient patients may be accrued in a reasonable time frame. The diseases that seem best to meet these criteria are breast cancer and small-cell lung cancer. In the former, the addition of cyclophosphamide to either CMF or CAF should be feasible, while in the later the combination of SR2508 with CAV would require a careful pilot study, because of the potential for overlapping neurotoxicity between vincristine and SR2508. It is hoped that a cooperative group trial in one of these two diseases will be feasible in the near future.

References

1. Sutherland RM. Cell and environment interactions in tumor microregions: the multicell spheroid model. Science 240:177–184, 1988.
2. Crabtree HG and Cramer W. The action of radium on cancer cells. II. Some factors determining the sensitivity of cancer cells to radium. Proc R Soc 113:238–250, 1933.
3. Kennedy KA, Teicher BA, Rockwell S, and Sartorelli AC. The hypoxic tumor cell: a target for selective cancer chemotherapy. Biochem Pharmacol 29:1–8, 1980.
4. Bush RS, Jenkin RDT, Allt WEC, et al. Definitive evidence for hypoxic cells influencing cure in cancer therapy. Br J Cancer 37 (Suppl. 111), 302–306, 1978.
5. Adams GE and Stratford IJ. Hypoxia-mediated nitro-heterocyclic drugs in the radio-and chemotherapy of cancer: an overview. Biochem Pharmacol 35, 71–76, 1986.
6. Tew KD and Clapper ML. Glutathione-S-transferases and anticancer drug resistance. In: Mechanisms of Drug Resistance in Cancer Cells, PV Woolley and KD Tew (eds). Academic Press, Orlando, FL, 1988, pp. 141–159.
7. Rice GC, Hoy C, and Schimke RT. Transient hypoxia enhances the frequency of dihydrofolate reductase gene amplification in Chinese hamster ovary cells. Proc Natl Acad Sci USA 83:5978–5982, 1986.
8. Sutherland RM, Heacock CS, Keng PC, Sciandra JJ, Seigrist ME, Smith HC, and Wilson RC. Hypoxia-induced enhanced synthesis of specific proteins, RNA and amplified DNA. Proc 6th Int Conf on Chemical Modifiers of Cancer Treatment, Paris, March 1988, #1–15.
9. Batist G, Tulpule A, Sinha BK, Katki AG, Myers CE, and Cowan KH. Overexpression of a novel anionic glutathione transferase in multidrug-resistance human breast cancer cells. J Biol Chem 261:15544–15549, 1986.
10. Sartorelli AC. Therapeutic attack of hypoxic cells of solid tumors. Presidential address. Cancer Res 48:775–778, 1988.
11. Guichard M, Chemical manipulations of tissue oxygenation for therapeutic benefit. Int J Radiat Oncol Biol Phys 16:1125–30, 1989.
12. Brown JM, Biaglow JE, Hall EJ, et al. Sensitizers and protectors to radiation and chemo-

therapeutic drugs. Cancer Treat Symposia 1:85–101, 1984.
13. Bleehen NM, Wiltshire CR, Plowman PN, et al. A randomized study of misonidazole and radiotherapy for grade 3 and 4 cerebral astrocytoma. Br J Cancer 43:436–442, 1981.
14. Sealy R, Williams A, Fridland S, et al. A report on misonidazole in a randomized trial in locally advanced head and neck cancer. Int J Radiat Oncol Biol Phys 8:339–342, 1982.
15. Brown JM and Workman P. Partition coefficient as a guide to the development of radiosensitizers which are less toxic than misonidazole. Radiat Res 82:171–190, 1980.
16. Bleehen NM, Freedman LS, and Stenning SP. A randomized study of CCNU with or without benznidazole in the treatment of recurrent grades 3 and 4 astrocytoma. Report to the Medical Research Council by the Brain Tumor Working Party. Int J Radiat Oncol Biol Phys 16:1077–1082, 1989.
17. Bleehen NM, Newman HFV, Maughan TS, and Workman, P. A multiple-dose study of the combined radiosensitizers Ro-03-8799 (pimonidazole) and SR 2508 (etanidazole). Int J Radiat Oncol Biol Phys 16:1093–1096, 1989.
18. Workman P. Pharmacokinetics of radiosensitizing agents. In: Pharmacokinetics of Anticancer Agents in Humans, Vol. 99. MM Ames, G Powis, and JS Kovach (eds). Elsevier, Amsterdam 1983; pp. 291–361.
19. Coleman CN, Wasserman TH, Urtasun RC, Halsey J, Hirst VK, Hancock S, and Phillips TL. Phase I trial of the hypoxic cell radiosensitizer SR 2508: the results of the five to six week drug schedule. Int J Radiat Oncol Biol Phys 12:1105–1108, 1986.
20. Clement JJ, Gorman MS, Wodinsky I, Catane R, and Johnson RK. Enhancement of antitumor activity of alkylating agents by the radiation sensitizer misonidazole. Cancer Res 40:4165–4172, 1980.
21. Rose CM, Millar JL, Peacock JH, Phelps TA, and Stephens TC. Differential enhancement of melphalan cytotoxicity in tumor and normal tissue by misonidazole. In: Radiation Sensitizers: Their Use in Clinical Management of Cancer, L Brady (ed). Masson Publishing, New York, 1980, p. 250.
22. Siemann DW. Modification of chemotherapy by nitroimidazoles. Int J Radiat Oncol Biol Phys 10:1585–1594, 1984.
23. Lam MP, Hirst DG, and Brown JM. The enhancing effect of misonidazole on the response of the RIF-1 tumor to cyclophosphamide. Br J Cancer 44:208–218, 1981.
24. Hirst DG, Hazlehurst JL, and Brown JM. Sensitization of normal and malignant tissues to cyclophosphamide by nitroimidazoles with different partition coefficients. Br J Cancer 49:33–42, 1984.
25. Siemann DW and Mulcahy RT. Sensitization of cancer chemotherapeutic agents by nitroheterocycles. Biochem Pharmacol 35:111–115, 1986.
26. Biaglow JE, Varnes ME, Roizen-Towle L, Clark EP, Epp ER, Astor MB, and Hall EJ. Biochemistry of reduction of nitroheterocycles. Biochem Pharmacol 35:77–90, 1986.
27. Kappus H. Overview of enzyme systems involved in bioreduction of drugs and in redox cycling. Biochem Pharmacol 35:1–6, 1986.
28. Walton MI, Wolf CR, and Workman P. Molecular enzymology of the reductive bioactivation of the hypoxic cells cytotoxins. Int J Radiat Oncol Biol Phys 16:983–986, 1989.
29. Ehlhardt WJ, Beaulieu BB, and Goldman P. Mammalian cell toxicity and bacterial mutagenicity of nitrosoimidazoles. Biochem Pharmacol 37:2603–2606, 1988.
30. Wong K-H and Agrawal KC. Role of nonprotein thiols in enzymatic reduction of 2-nitroimidazoles. Biochem Pharmacol 37:473–479, 1988.
31. Varghese AJ and Whitmore GF. Identification of a reactive glutathione conjugate as a metabolite of SR2508 in CHO cells. Int J Radiat Oncol Biol Phys 1986; 12:1223–1226.
32. Kumar KS and Weiss JF. Inhibition of glutathione peroxidase and glutathione transferase in mouse liver by misonidazole. Biochem Pharmacol 35:3143–3146, 1986.
33. Taylor YC, Evans JW, and Brown JM. Mechanism of sensitization of Chinese hamster ovary cells to melphalan by hypoxic treatment with misonidazole. Cancer Res 43:3175–3181, 1983.

34. Hinchcliffe M, McNally NJ, and Stratford MRL. The effect of radiosensitizers on the pharmacokinetics of melphalan and cyclophosphamide in the mouse. Br J Cancer 48:375–383, 1983.
35. Tutsch K, Mulcahy RT, Trump D, et al. Phase I clinical and pharmacokinetic trial of SR 2508 and cyclophosphamide administered by short infusion. Proc Am Assoc Cancer Res 30:241, 1989.
36. O'Dwyer, PJ, LaCreta FP, Walczak J, Hoffman J, Langer C, Tew K, and Comis R. SR 2508/cyclophosphamide: clinical and pharmacokinetic results at high doses. Proc Am Assoc Cancer Res 30:243, 1989.
37. Workman P and Brown JM. Structure-pharmacokinetic relationships for misonidazole analogues in mice. Cancer Chemother Pharmacol 6:39–49, 1981.
38. Flockhart IR, Large P, Troup D, Malcolm SL, and Marten, TR. Pharmacokinetic and metabolic studies of the hypoxic cell radiosensitizer misonidazole. Xenobiotica 8:97–105, 1978.
39. Josephy PD, Palcic B, and Skarsgard LD. Reduction of misonidazole and its derivatives by xanthine oxidase. Biochem Pharmacol 30:849–853, 1981.
40. Koch RL, Beaulieu BB Jr., and Goldman P. Role of the intestinal flora in the metabolism of misonidazole. Biochem Pharmacol 29:3281–3284, 1980.
41. Rao DN and Mason RP. Generation of nitro radical anions of some 5-nitrofurans, 2- and 5-nitroimidazoles by rat hepatocytes. Biochem Pharmacol 37:2907–2913, 1988.
42. Rauth AM, McClelland RA, Michaels HB, and Battistella R. The oxygen dependence of the reduction of nitroimidazoles is a radiolytic model system. Int J Radiat Oncol Biol Phys 10:1323–1326, 1984.
43. White RAS, Workman P, and Brown JM. The pharmacokinetics and tumor and neural tissue penetrating properties of SR 2508 in the dog: hydrophilic radiosensitizers potentially less toxic than misonidazole. Radiation Res 84:542–561, 1980.
44. Workman P. Micropharmacokinetics of chemical modifiers. Int J Radiat Oncol Biol Phys 16:897–906, 1989.
45. Brown JM. Clinical trials of radiosensitizers: what should we expect? Int J Radiat Oncol Biol Phys 10:425–429, 1984.
46. Dische S. Chemical sensitizers for hypoxic cells: decade of experience in clinical radiotherapy. Radiother Oncol 3:97–115, 1985.
47. Ohno T, Saeki T, Urano M, Watanabe I, and Shikita M. Mode of radiosensitization of hypoxic cells by furylfuramide. J Radiat Res 18:275–279, 1977.
48. Russell KJ, Brown DM, Yu N, Conley F, and Luck E. Intratumoral diffusion-limited cytotoxic chemotherapy for localized potentiation of radiation: pre-clinical pharmacokinetic and biodistribution studies in *in vivo* trials of efficacy. Int J Radiat Oncol Biol Phys 13(Suppl 1):171, 1987.
49. Brown DQ, Unger EC, Beck AC, and Needleman PF. Intratumoral injection of the radiosensitizer SR-2508 to sensitize hypoxic radiation resistant tumors. Int J Radiat Oncol Biol Phys.
50. Brown DQ and Cirruci LM. Tumor retention and plasma levels of intratumorally injected SR-2508. Proceedings of the Radiation Research Society.
51. LaCreta FP, Helfand SC, and Evans SM. Pharmacokinetics of the radiosensitizer SR-2508 following intravenous and intratumoral administration in cats. Proc Am Assoc Cancer Res 30:2147, 1989.
52. Coleman CN, Bump EA, and Kramer RR. Chemical modifiers of cancer treatment. J Clin Oncol 6:709–733, 1988.
53. Coleman CN, Halsey J, Cox RS, et al. Relationship between the neurotoxicity of the hypoxic cell radiosensitizer SR 2508 and the pharmacokinetic profile. Cancer Res 47:319–311, 1987.
54. Roberts JT, Bleehan NM, Walton MI, and Workman P. A clinical phase I toxicity study of Ro 03-8799: plasma, urine, tumor and normal brain pharmacokinetics. Br J Radiol 59:107–116, 1986.

55. Honess DJ, Wasserman TH, Workman P, Ward R, and Bleehan NM. Additivity of radio-sensitization by the combination of SR 2508 (etanidazole) and Ro 03-8799 (pimonidazole) in a murine tumor system. Int J Radiat Oncol Biol Phys 15:671–675, 1988.
56. Lai GM, Ozols RF, Young RC, and Hamilton TC. Effects of glutathione and DNA repair in cisplatin-resistant human ovarian cancer cell line. J Natl Cancer Inst 81:535–539, 1989.

4. Folate antimetabolites inhibitory to *de novo* purine synthesis

Richard G. Moran

Introduction

The discovery of the activity of methotrexate (figure 1) for the treatment of human cancers in the early 1950s prompted the search for other folate analogs that were more active than methotrexate or, at least, that had different properties than this important folate antimetabolite. After 40 years of preclinical and clinical investigation, methotrexate is still in clinical use and still represents the only folate analog in widespread therapeutic application for the treatment of cancers. This is the case, in spite of the fact that thousands of folate analogs have been made and studied in the interim and that the potential of folate antimetabolites as therapeutic agents is established. Of course, the pharmaceutical promise for a new class of folate antimetabolites also continues to be high, given the central nature of the folate-dependent enzymes in processes required for any proliferative cell population.

There are at least 11 folate-dependent enzymes that are expressed in rapidly dividing mammalian cell populations (figure 2). It appears that *all* of these enzymes are essential for the survival of mammalian neoplastic or normal stem cells and, hence, that they each represent a new potential target for cancer chemotherapy. Until recently, the only enzyme of this pathway for which potent inhibitors was available was dihydrofolate reductase (DHFR). In 1980, Jones and his colleagues at the Institute for Cancer Research in England identified 10-propargyl-5,8-dideazafolate (CB 3717, PDDF) (figure 1) as a potent inhibitor of thymidylate synthase [1,2]. This observation was of fundamental importance to the field, because it established the precedent that folate analogs inhibitory to thymidylate synthase were alternatives to the fluoropyrimidines for cancer chemotherapy. In fact, such folate-based chemotherapy targeted at thymidylate synthase circumvents some of the major factors (such as low tumor cell folate co-factors and high accumulation of deoxyuridylate) that limit tumor cell kill by precursors of 5-fluoro-2′-deoxyuridine-5′-monophosphate [3]. More generally, CB 3717 furnished a tremendous stimulus for the development of folate antimetabolites inhibitory to enzymes other than DHFR, due not only to the

Franco M. Muggia (ed.), NEW DRUGS, CONCEPTS AND RESULTS IN CANCER CHEMOTHERAPY.
 ISBN 0–7923–1253–8

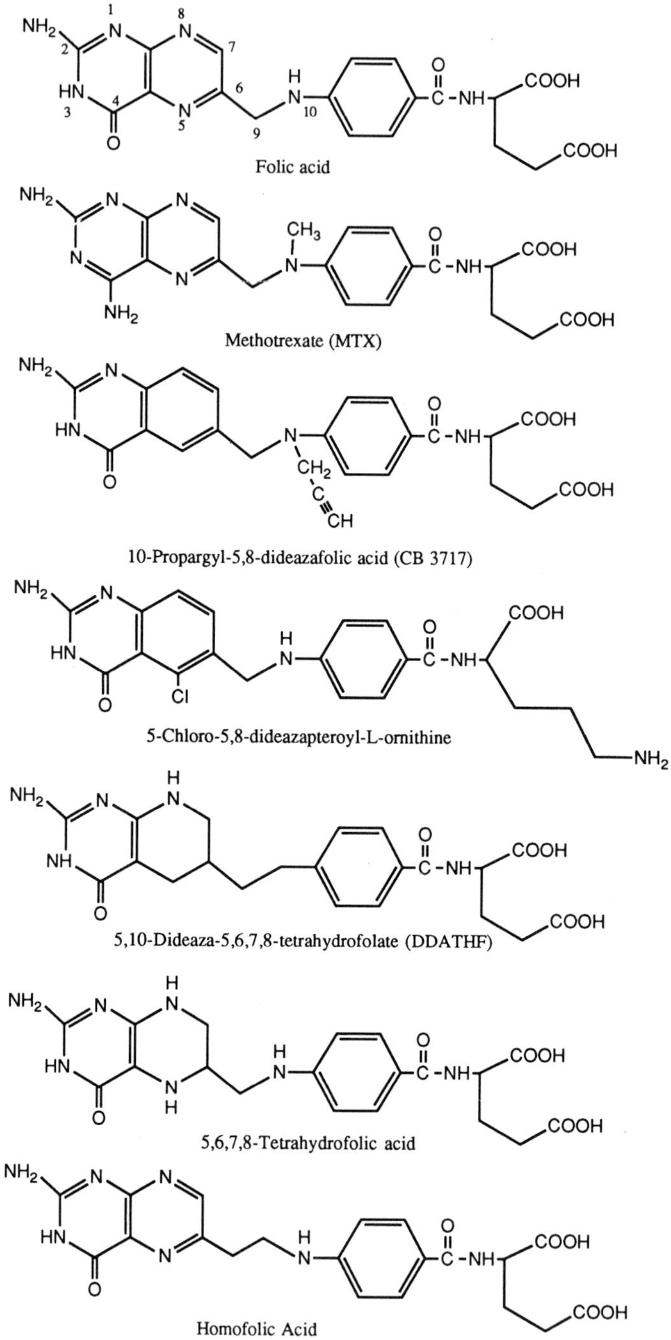

Figure 1. A comparison of the structures of landmark folate antimetabolites with that of folic acid and of tetrahydrofolate.

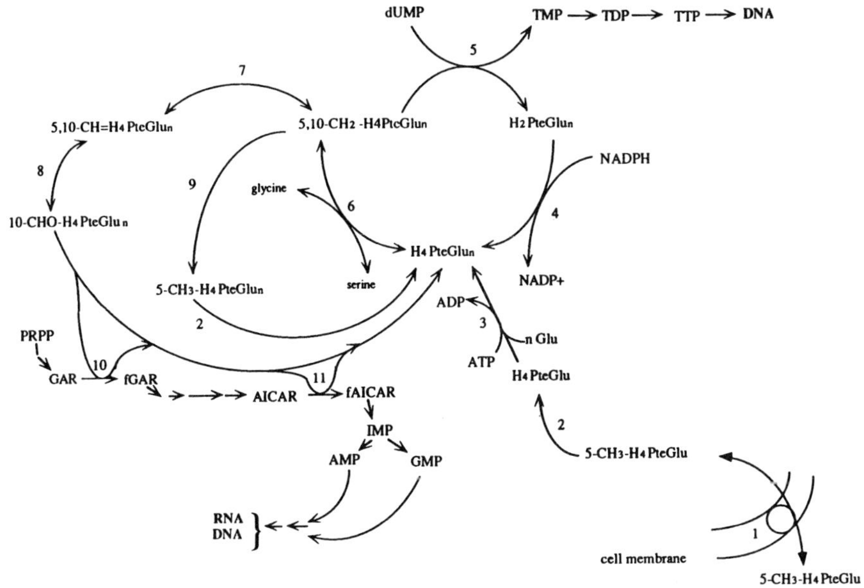

Figure 2. Enzymatic interconversions in the folate pathway. These reactions are catalyzed by (1) the high-affinity reduced-folate carrier-mediated transport system; (2) methionine synthase, a methylcobalamin-dependent enzyme that salvages homocysteine from the S-adenosyl methionine pathway with the resynthesis of methionine; (3) the conversion of the tetrahydrofolyl monoglutamates to polyglutamate forms by folylpoly-γ-glutamate synthetase (FPGS); (4) the resynthesis of tetrahydrofolates by dihydrofolate reductase after loss as dihydrofolate during thymidylate synthesis; (5) thymidylate synthase; (6) serine hydroxymethyltransferase; (7) 5,10-methylenetetrahydrofolate dehydrogenase; (8) 5,10-methenyltetrahydrofolate cyclohydrolase; (9) 5,10-methylenetetrahydrofolate reductase; (10) glycinamide ribonucleotide formyltransferase (GARFT); (11) aminoimidazole carboxamide ribonucleotide formyltransferase (AICARFT).

theoretical interest in this compound, but also to the fact that it showed activity against human disease, even in a phase 1 patient population [4–6]. More recently, the first reports appeared of potent inhibitors of the critical folate-dependent enzyme, folylpoly-γ-glutamate synthetase (FPGS). The structure of the most potent of this series reported to date, 5-chloro-5,8-dideazapteroyl-L-ornithine [7] is shown in figure 1. This advance was the result of the observation by Shane that a derivative of tetrahydrofolic acid in which the glutamic acid side chain was replaced by L-ornithine was a moderately potent inhibitor of FPGS [8]. Shane's finding was quickly followed up by several groups [7, 8–10], and the activity of the lead compound was improved by second-generation compounds in which the tetrahydropteridine moiety of tetrahydropteroyl-L-ornithine was replaced by heterocyclic rings that bound tighter to the active site of FPGS than did the pteridine moiety. Unfortunately, the utility of 5-chloro-5,8-dideazapteroyl-L-ornithine and all of the analogs of this series appears limited to biochemical studies because of the poor membrane penetration of these analogs

[10, 11]. A definition of the suitability of FPGS as a target for chemotherapy [12] will have to await folate analogs or other new inhibitors that are freely membrane permeable. A third major advance was introduced in 1985 with the report of a novel folate antimetabolite that was inactive as an inhibitor of DHFR [13] but was a potent inhibitor of *de novo* purine synthesis [14]. This compound, 5,10-dideaza-5,6,7,8-tetrahydrofolate (figure 1), aroused immediate interest and has proven to be the prototype of a new class of folate analogs of substantial theoretical importance and of potential clinical utility. The purpose of this chapter is to outline what is currently known about this compound and other promising antimetabolites of this class.

Early folate inhibitors of *de novo* purine synthesis: Tetrahydrohomofolate

Homofolic acid is the trivial name given to the folic acid analog that has one more methylene group between the 2-amino-4-oxo-pteridine ring and p-aminobenzoylglutamic acid than is found in the folic acid molecule (figure 1). Tetrahydrohomofolic acid was originally found to be a potent inhibitor of thymidylate synthase in the course of experiments that utilized *E. coli* enzyme [15]. When it was found that homofolic acid was reduced to tetrahydrohomofolic acid by dihydrofolate reductase, it appeared that an ideal case of the concept of 'collateral sensitivity' had been discovered [15, 16]. Thus, it was well known that tumor cells can become resistant to methotrexate by fixing multiple copies of the dihydrofolate reductase gene in the genome, either as double-minute chromosomes or as stably integrated homogeneously staining regions [17–20]. This excessive dosage of a transcriptional active gene for dihydrofolate reductase results in an increased content of this enzyme in tumor cells and resistance to methotrexate [17–20]. This higher cellular activity of dihydrofolate reductase should activate homofolate to tetrahydrohomofolate more rapidly in tumor cells that are resistant to methotrexate by virtue of gene amplification. Mead and his colleagues subsequently reported [21, 22] that some experimental tumors made resistant to methotrexate *in vivo* showed collateral sensitivity to homofolate derivatives when tested *in vivo*. Others did not find this to be the case with cultured tumor cell lines [23, 24], an experimental system more amenable to a test of this hypothesis. In retrospect, at least one aspect of the original concept was subsequently proven incorrect when it was found that, although tetrahydrohomofolate was an inhibitor of bacterial thymidylate synthase [15], it was almost inactive against thymidylate synthase from a mammalian tumor [25–27], as are the polyglutamate forms of tetrahydrohomofolate [27]. The inactivity or very low activity of polyglutamate forms of tetrahydrohomofolate for mammalian thymidylate synthase is even more remarkable in view of the fact that polyglutamates of CB 3717 are up to 100 times more potent than CB 3717 itself. Hence, one can surmise that tetrahydrohomofolate is indeed inactive against mammalian thymidylate synthase if the amplifying effects of polyglutamation do not result in enzyme inhibition. This situation illustrated an interesting and important difference between bacterial and mammalian thymidylate synthases: in spite of ~55% identity in amino acid sequence between mouse and *L. casei* thymidylate synthases [28, 29], inhibitors of one enzyme could not be assumed to inhibit the other. On the other hand, given that homofolates had been demonstrated to be active antitumor agents in vivo [21, 22], it was clear that another step in tumor cell folate metabolism was sensitive to these compounds.

Classical studies by Hakala [30] rekindled a broad interest in the homofolate derivatives. Contrary to previous ideas on the action of the homofolates, Hakala found that inclusion of thymidine in cell culture medium had no effect on the growth inhibition caused by homofolate or tetrahydrohomofolate to mouse Sarcoma 180 (S-180) cells. However, a source of preformed purines, such as hypoxanthine, virtually eliminated the effects of homofolate. This was a clear indication that homofolic acid had little or no effect on thymidylate synthase, but rather inhibited cell growth by virtue of an effect on purine synthesis. Cellular studies by Divekar and Hakala [31] suggested that exposure of S-180 cells to homofolic acid resulted in inhibition of glycinamide ribonucleotide formyltransferase (GARFT). Further studies in several laboratories [32–34] confirmed that inhibition of tumor cell growth by any of several homofolate derivatives was due to effects on purine synthesis.

With the knowledge that the homofolates are antimetabolites of *de novo* purine synthesis, it seems likely that the ultimate antiproliferative form of the homofolates would be an antimetabolite of 10-formyltetrahydrofolate, the folate cofactor form used as a cosubstrate by both of the folate-dependent enzymes of *de novo* purine synthesis. As a result, 11-formyl tetrahydrohomofolate and 5,11-methenyltetrahydrohomofolate [34, 35], and 5-formyl-tetrahydrohomofolate [32], were synthesized and studied as inhibitors of purine biosynthesis. Slieker and Benkovic found that 5,11-methenyltetrahydrohomofolate inhibited the growth of hamster cells with a pattern that suggested aminoimidazole carboxamide ribonucleotide formyltransferase (AICARFT) as a target [34]. However, 11-formyltetrahydrohomofolate was an inhibitor of chicken liver GARFT with a K_i of ~1 μM [34]. 5-Formyltetrahydrohomofolate was first synthesized in the author's laboratory using a direct condensation of formic acid with (6S)-tetrahydrohomofolate that was promoted by carbodiimides [32]. This reaction was subsequently adapted by others [36] to a 'one-pot' synthesis from homofolate without intermediate purification of the reduced product with less than adequate results; several products were obtained [37]. Nevertheless, 5-formyltetrahydrohomofolate, as originally prepared, was pure and had several characteristics that suggested it to be a preferable form of the homofolate compounds:

1. It was very stable in neutral aqueous phase.

2. It presumably could be metabolized to 11-formyltetrahydrohomofolate by a single-step reaction.
3. It was originally thought that 5-formyltetrahydrohomofolate should be a good substrate for FPGS, like 5-formyltetrahydrofolate, and in contrast to the poor utilization of 5-methyltetrahydrofolate (and 5-methyltetrahydrohomofolate) by FPGS [38, 39].

When these assumptions were directly tested, 5-formyltetrahydrohomofolate was found to be an exceptionally poor substrate for mouse liver FPGS [32]; this has never been adequately explained.

The antiproliferative effects of 5-formyltetrahydrohomofolate, like those of 5,11-methenyltetrahydrohomofolate, were not affected by the presence of aminoimidazolecarboxamide in the growth medium [32, 33]. This has been taken as evidence that the growth-limiting events with both compounds are inhibition of AICARFT. This observation is not consistent with studies on the isolated folate-dependent transformylases of purine synthesis. These results indicated inhibition of GARFT by tetrahydrohomofolate and its polyglutamates, with little or no effect of these compounds on AICARFT [26, 27].

The overwhelming limitation of the homofolate analogs is their low potency. Thus, even under conditions of continuous exposure of tumor cells in culture, concentrations in the range of 2–50 μM were required to exert an antiproliferative effect on a spectrum of tumor cell lines (table 1) [41]. This is also reflected by the outcome of a phase 1 clinical trial on (6R,S)5-methyltetrahydrohomofolate, which was terminated when dose escalation to 5 g/m^2 failed to produce either antitumor effects or any serious host toxicity [42]. This low potency seems explained by the fact that, in contrast to what is seen with deazatetrahydrofolates (see below), the homofolates are very poor substrates for folylpoly-γ-glutamate synthetase from mouse [32, 43] and hog liver [38].

5,10-Dideaza-5,6,7,8-tetrahydrofolate (DDATHF)

Early studies

The synthesis of four folate analogs was reported in 1985 in which the nitrogens at the 5 and 10 positions of the aminopterin, folic acid, tetrahydroaminopterin, and tetrahydrofolate molecules had been replaced by carbons [13]. All four of these compounds were intrinsically interesting because the 5 and 10 nitrogens are the site of attachment during the folate-dependent one-carbon transfers (figures 1 and 2), but one of the four immediately demonstrated some intriguing biochemical properties. That compound was 5,10-dideaza-5,6,7,8-tetrahydrofolate, or DDATHF. DDATHF and 5,10-dideazatetrahydroaminopterin were originally synthesized as inhibitors of thymidylate synthase, but both compounds proved to be virtually

Table 1. Inhibition of the growth of mammalian tumor cells by homofolate derivatives.

Compound	Cell Line	IC50 (μM)	Ref.
Homofolate	S-180	15	30
	S-180	7	23
	L1210	17	32
	Manca	6	27
11-Formylhomofolate	HKSV28	14	34
Tetrahydrohomofolate	S-180	20	30
5-Methyltetrahydrohomofolate	L1210	5.6	32
	Manca	8	27
5,11-Methenyltetrahydrohomofolate	HKSV28	4	34
5-Formyltetrahydrohomofolate	L1210	5.0	32
	MCF-7	2.0	33
(6S)5-Formyltetrahydrohomofolate	L1210	1.7	32
8-Deazahomofolate	L1210	88	40
8-Deazatetrahydrohomofolate	L1210	36	40

inactive against this enzyme [13, 44]. 5,10-Dideazatetrahydroaminopterin, although a very cytotoxic compound [13], has been largely ignored since the report of its synthesis. DDATHF would have suffered the same fate had it not been for two clear signals of its potential importance: it was a superb substrate for folylpolyglutamate synthetase, and it had an unusual pattern of inhibition of the growth of tumor cells in culture at very low concentrations [14, 44, 45]. Although there are now a number of examples of synthetic folate compounds whose activities as substrates for FPGS rival or exceed those of the naturally occurring folates [7, 8, 46–49], that was not the case in 1984, and the efficiency of utilization of DDATHF by this enzyme was striking (figure 3). It is particularly impressive that several of the second-generation analogs of DDATHF, for instance, 5-deazatetrahydrofolate, are much more efficiently utilized as a substrate by FPGS (figure 3B) [48]. The inhibition of leukemic cell growth by DDATHF was made much more exciting by the virtual inactivity of this compound against the two 'classical' targets of folate antimetabolites, dihydrofolate reductase (E.C.1.5.1.3) and thymidylate synthase (E.C.2.1.1.45) [13, 44]. As a result, a series of cell culture experiments was performed to determine the mechanism of the anti-proliferative activity of DDATHF [14, 44]. The results of the first experiment, which are reproduced in figure 4, indicated that the presence of thymidine in the culture medium did not alter the growth-inhibitory potency of DDATHF but that, in the presence of a precursor of purines such as hypoxanthine, DDATHF was without effect on the tumor cells at any concentration tested. From these earliest studies, it was clear that DDATHF is an antimetabolite that is inhibitory to *de novo* purine synthesis and is two orders of magnitude more potent than the homofolates.

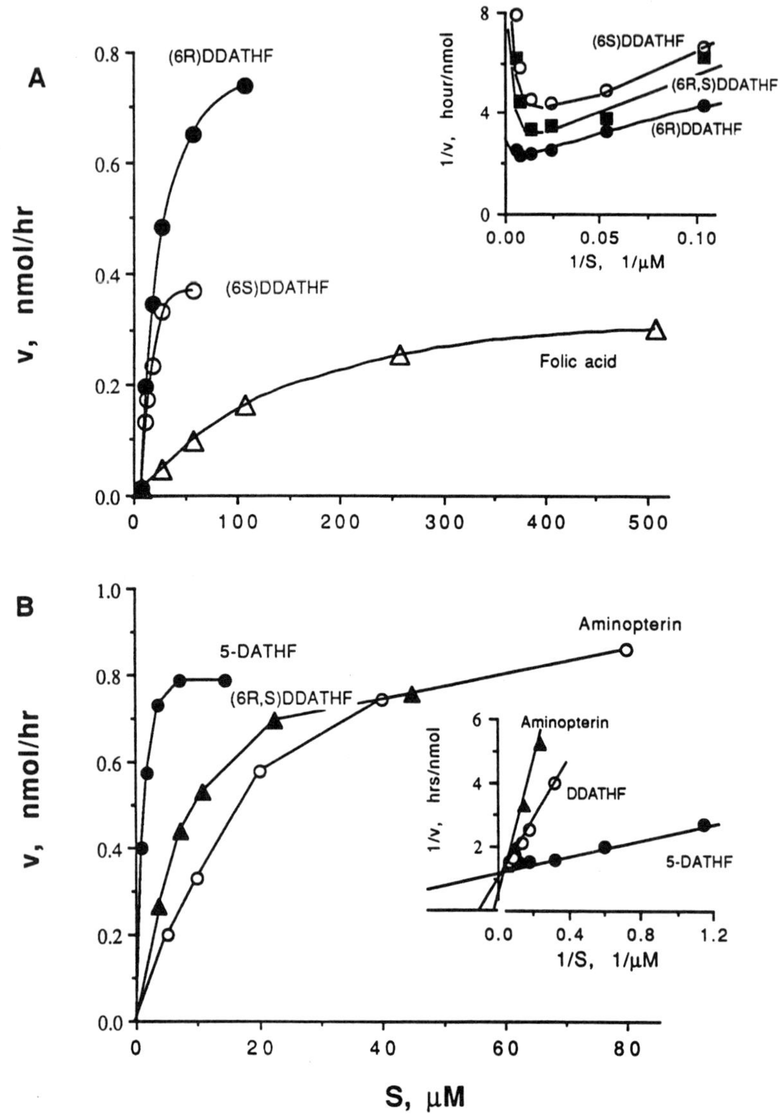

Figure 3. The activity of DDATHF as a substrate for folylpolyglutamate synthetase. (A) Rate of reaction as a function of the concentration of each of the diastereomers differing in chirality about carbon 6. Folic acid is used as an internal standard. Note the equivalent K_m values for the two isomers but the distinctly higher V_{max} of the 6R isomer. The inset demonstrates substrate inhibition with the 6S but not the 6R isomer. (B) A comparison of the concentration dependence of the FPGS reaction *in vitro* with aminopterin, DDATHF, and 5-deazatetrahydrofolate 5-DATHF. The inset demonstrates that aminopterin, which is usually thought of as an excellent substrate for this enzyme, is inefficiently utilized when compared to either DDATHF or 5-DATHF. Mouse liver enzyme was used in these experiments.

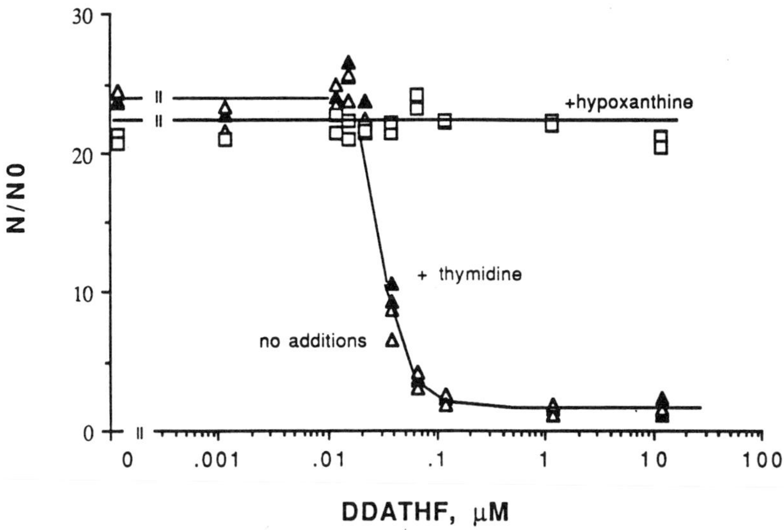

Figure 4. Prevention of the growth inhibition of DDATHF by purines. The amount of growth of cultures of mouse leukemia L1210 cells that occurred during 72 hours of incubation with increasing concentrations of (6R,S) DDATHF is shown either in basal medium supplemented with dialyzed fetal calf serum or with the addition of 5.6 μM thymidine or 32 μM hypoxanthine.

Site of action of DDATHF

De novo purine synthesis consists of 10 sequential enzymatic reactions (figure 5). Two of these, glycinamide ribonucleotide formyltransferase (E.C.2.1.2.2, GARFT) and aminoimidazolecarboxamide ribonucleotide formyltransferase (E.C.2.1.2.3, AICARFT), are folate dependent and catalyze the transfer of the 10-formyl group from (6R)10-formyltetrahydrofolate to a primary amino group. A critical question during the early phases of investigation of DDATHF was whether this compound was selectively active against one of these two enzymes. Three lines of evidence led us to the conclusion that GARFT was the predominant, if not the exclusive, target for DDATHF cytotoxicity [14, 44]. The first information to resolve this question was that aminoimidazolecarboxamide (AICA) protected L1210 cells from DDATHF. As shown in figure 5, AICA is activated to aminoimidazolecarboxamide ribonucleotide, and hence, is capable of protecting cells from any inhibitor of steps in this pathway prior to AICARFT, such as GARFT, but would not be expected to substantially affect the potency of an inhibitor of AICARFT. Inclusion of AICA in cell culture medium prevented the growth-inhibitory effects of DDATHF for both mouse L1210 and CEM human leukemia cells [44]. A more direct avenue of evidence to this point was suggested by an experiment previously used by Henderson [50] and by Divekar and Hakala [31] to study early events in *de novo* purine synthesis.

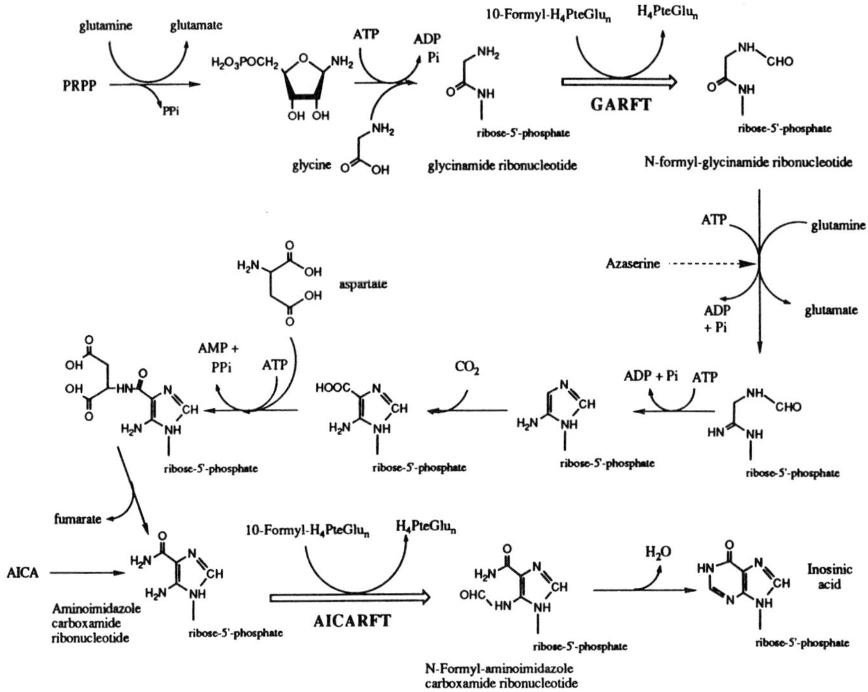

Figure 5. Reaction of the *de novo* synthesis of the purine ring. The two folate-dependent reactions, catalyzed by GARFT and AICARFT, are denoted by open arrows. The principal site of inhibition of this pathway by azaserine is shown, as are the sites of entry of (^{14}C) glycine and AICA into the pathway.

These groups had labeled early intermediates in the purine synthesis pathway with ^{14}C-glycine and studied the accumulation of ^{14}C as formylglycinamide ribonucleotide after poisoning *de novo* purine synthesis with the glutamine antagonist azaserine (figure 5). This technique was ideal for the study of DDATHF, and we used it to demonstrate that DDATHF interfered with the accumulation of ^{14}C-glycine as ^{14}C-formylglycinamide ribonucleotide in the presence of azaserine (figure 6) [44]. This approach also revealed that the concentration dependence of inhibition of formylglycinamide accumulation by DDATHF was superimposable on the dose response of growth inhibition caused by DDATHF in L1210 cells (figure 6). Although these two lines of cellular evidence were very convincing, the most direct evidence for inhibition of GARFT by DDATHF has come from studies in cell-free enzyme systems. A report from another laboratory [51] indicated that DDATHF inhibited GARFT activity in crude cytosols of mammalian cells, as did early studies in our laboratory [unpublished results]. Subsequently, we reported definitive kinetic experiments using pure enzyme [45] that demonstrated that DDATHF was a potent inhibitor of mouse L1210 cell GARFT; inhibition was competitive with the folate substrate. This was

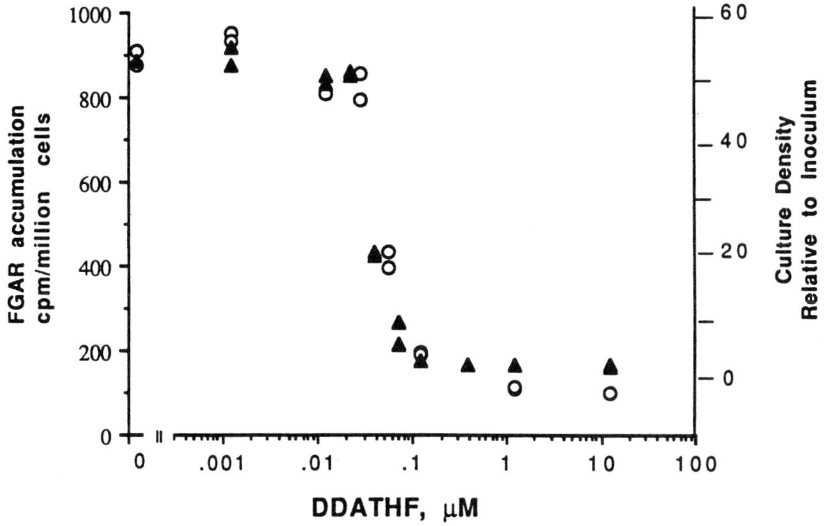

Figure 6. Correlation of the concentrations of DDATHF that inhibit cell growth (▲) with those that block the synthesis of N-formylglycinamide ribonucleotide (○) in mouse L1210 leukemia cells. For details, see reference 44.

the first data that allowed a meaningful assessment of the strength of the binding of DDATHF to GARFT.

Stereochemistry of DDATHF

The DDATHF structure has two centers of asymmetry, the α-carbon of the glutamic acid side chain and the 6-position of the heterocyclic ring (figure 1). Because the original synthesis [13] proceeded through intermediates that incorporated L-glutamic acid as a side chain but through a non-stereoselective chemical reduction of the pyridopyrimidine ring, the resultant compound was a mixture of two diastereomers, differing in orientation about the 6-carbon. These two chemically distinct compounds were separated by Dr. Chuan Shih of Eli Lilly Research Laboratories using fractional crystallization, and also by chiral high-performance liquid chromatography [45]. Subsequently, the diastereomer of DDATHF that had the same orientation of the 6-H as the naturally-occurring tetrahydrofolate compounds was shown to have the 6-R absolute configuration. This assignment was based on an unambiguous chemical synthesis of each diastereomer from precursors of known stereochemistry by Drs. Barnett and Wilson, also of Eli Lilly Research Laboratories [52]. The availability of these compounds allowed a direct assessment of which of these isomers was responsible for the biological activity of this compound. We were very surprised to find that both the 6-S and 6-R diastereomers of DDATHF not only had activity against mammalian tumor cells in culture, but also, for the L1210 leukemia cell, the

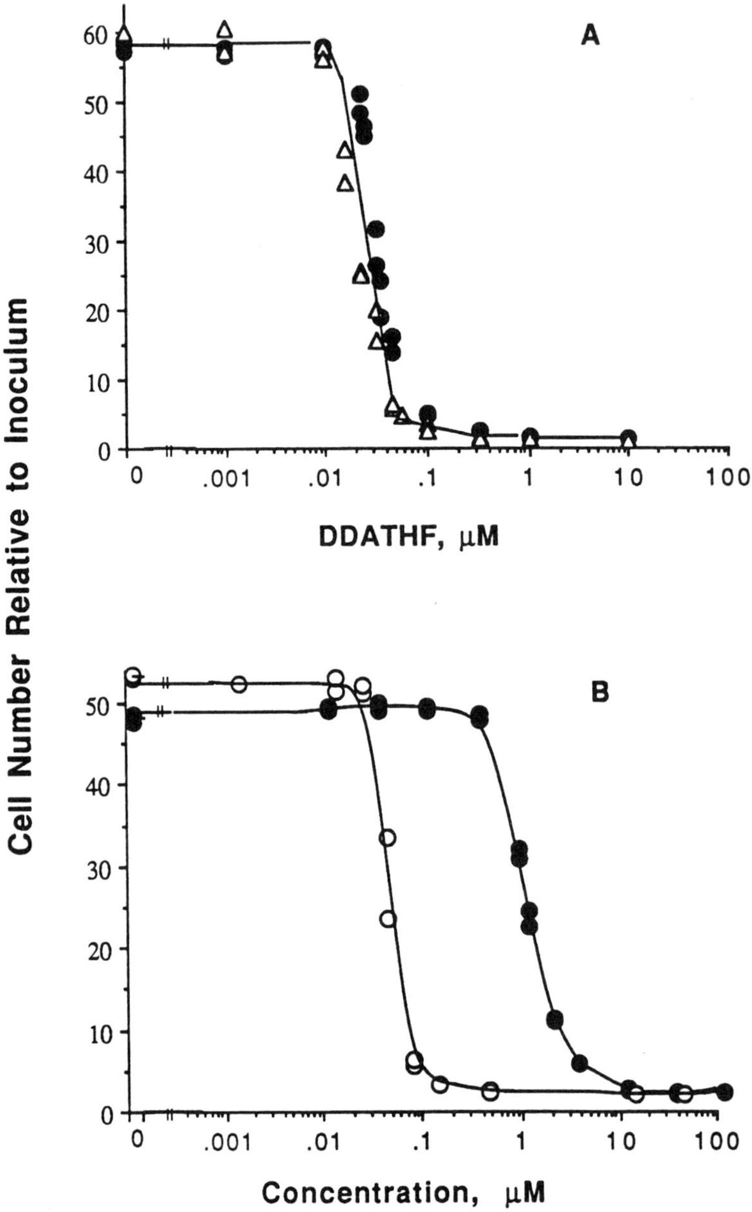

Figure 7. Inhibition of the growth of L1210 cells by the 6R (△) and 6S (●) diastereomers of DDATHF (A) and by (6R,S) DDATHF (○) and (6R,S) 5,10-dideazatetrahydropteroyl-L-aspartate (●) (B). Cultures were continuously exposed to the indicated concentration of compounds during a 72-hour incubation at 37°C. The results shown represent data from a single experiment; each symbol is a single culture. Even the small difference seen in (A) between (6R) and (6S) diastereomers was less significant when the results of multiple experiments were averaged. For details, see reference 45.

growth inhibition caused by (6R) and by (6S)DDATHF was virtually identical (figure 7A) [45]. As the individual steps involved in the action of DDATHF were studied with the individual diastereomers, it was found that the activity of both compounds as substrates for FPGS from both mouse and human tissue, the activity against pure L1210 GARFT, and the reversal of each diastereomer by 5-formyltetrahydrofolate were nearly identical [45]. This was remarkable and indicated a level of stereoselectivity much lower than would have been expected *a priori*. However, literature precedent existed that this might be the case. Thus, prior studies on enzyme of both bacterial [53] and murine [54] sources indicated that (6-R)10-formyltetrahydrofolate is the substrate for GARFT, but that the unnatural diastereomer is a potent inhibitor and, hence, can bind to these proteins. Likewise, previous studies on FPGS of mouse and rat liver origins indicated that both (6R) and (6S) diastereomers of tetrahydrofolate could be utilized as substrates [55, 56]. In addition, both diastereomers of 5-formyltetrahydrofolate were reported to be substrates for mouse liver FPGS [56]. However, previous studies on FPGS had indicated a major difference in the kinetics of the reaction with natural and unnatural diastereomers. The differences we found with the diastereomers of DDATHF were more subtle: the diastereomers with the C-6 configuration opposite to the orientation of that found in the natural tetrahydrofolates demonstrated substrate inhibition for mouse liver FPGS, while (6-R)DDATHF did not [45]. Insights into this lack of stereoselectivity of DDATHF have evolved from an unexpected source: structure-activity relationships for inhibition of GARFT and for substrate activity with FPGS (see below).

Biochemical steps in the cytotoxicity of DDATHF

Passage through the plasma membrane. Convincing indirect evidence suggests that DDATHF is translocated into mammalian cells primarily by the same high-affinity carrier-mediated transport system responsible for transport of reduced folates and of methotrexate into cells. Thus, DDATHF interferes with the transport of ^{3}H-methotrexate in both CEM human [57] and L1210 mouse leukemic cells [51, 58]. The concentrations of DDATHF that interfered with MTX transport were comparable to the K_t for methotrexate. L1210 and CEM cell lines resistant to MTX by virtue of a defect in the reduced folate transport system were reported to be cross-resistant to DDATHF [58, 59]. This strongly implies that entry of DDATHF into tumor cells is predominantly mediated by the high-affinity, reduced folate carrier system but, of course, does not rule out the involvement of other proteins in this translocation.

Polyglutamation. Both diastereomers of DDATHF are efficiently utilized by FPGS from mouse liver and from human leukemic cells [45]. It has recently been reported [60] that human leukemic cells accumulate substantial quantities of DDATHF polyglutamates, with a total of up to seven glutamates per mole of heterocycle. As has been shown to be the case for all other classes of folate and antifolate polyglutamates [61–63], the polyglutamate derivatives of DDATHF were retained in tumor cells under conditions in which DDATHF effluxed into the medium [60]. The critical observation was also made recently that 5-formyltetrahydrofolate interfered with the biosynthesis of polyglutamates of DDATHF in tumor cells under conditions in which the antiproliferative effects of DDATHF were prevented [64]. This implies that polyglutamation of DDATHF is central to the development of the cytotoxicity of DDATHF, as does the recent observation by Pizzorno and his colleagues [65] that CEM cell lines resistant to DDATHF are deficient in FPGS activity.

Inhibition of GARFT. Early studies on DDATHF indicated that GARFT activity became limiting to *de novo* purine synthesis in mouse and human leukemic cells exposed to $\geqslant 3 \times 10^{-8}$ M drug (table 2) (see above). Subsequently, it was shown that DDATHF and many of its structural analogs inhibited pure GARFT *in vitro* [45, 67]. Inhibition was competitive with the folate substrate and noncompetitive with glycinamide ribonucleotide [45, 67]. Surprisingly, DDATHF was not very potent (K_i = 0.03–0.12 μM) when compared with other similarly cytotoxic compounds, e.g., methotrexate, which often inhibits dihydrofolate reductases with a K_i in the range of 10^{-12} to 10^{-9} M [68]. Two factors seem to explain this apparent discrepancy. First, the polyglutamate derivatives of DDATHF are much more potent inhibitors of GARFT than is DDATHF itself [67]. Second, the abundance of GARFT in at least some tumor cells is equivalent to a cytosolic concentration of enzyme approaching 1 μM [67]. Thus, with the concentration of both enzyme and polyglutamate forms of inhibitor in a concentration range >1000 times higher than the K_i for the drug-enzyme interaction, the system would clearly be in the zone C behavior described by Strauss and Goldstein [69]. Werkheiser [70] defined this situation as *stoichiometric* inhibition, in recognition of the fact that it is the ratio of K_i to the enzyme concentration that determines the tightness of target-drug interactions.

AICARTF. Cellular experiments had suggested that the action of the 6R and 6S diastereomers of DDATHF differed only in detail in L1210 mouse leukemia cells [45]. There was a suggestion, however, that exposure of cells to high concentrations of (6R)DDATHF resulted in some inhibition of AICARFT, whereas this effect was not seen with (6S)DDATHF. These conclusions were originally drawn on the basis that, in the presence of preformed purines such as hypoxanthine, inhibition of cell growth was not seen at any concentration of either diastereomer studied, while in AICA-supplemented medium, high concentrations of (6S)DDATHF (but not (6R)DDATHF) inhibited tumor cell growth [45]. Recently, a preliminary report by Pizzorno et al. [60] indicated direct evidence for activity of higher polyglutamates of DDATHF as inhibitors of purified AICARFT

Table 2. Inhibition of the growth of mammalian tumor cells by deazatetrahydrofolates.

Compound	Cell Line	IC50 (μM)	Ref.
5,10-Dideazatetrahydrofolate	L1210	0.028	12, 44
	L1210	0.057	51
	L1210	0.225[a]	57
	CEM	0.008	12, 44
	CEM	0.023	58
	CEM	0.02	46
	H35	0.220[a]	66
5-Deazatetrahydrofolate	CEM	0.010	48
10-Methyl-5-deazatetrahydrofolate	CEM	0.040	48
10-Methyl-5,10-dideazatetrahydrofolate	L1210	0.050	51
10-Ethyl-5,10-dideazatetrahydrofolate	L1210	0.035	51
5-Deazaacyclotetrahydrofolate	Detriot 98	0.11	74
	L	0.088	74
	A 427	0.043	74
	MCF-7	0.037	74
	WiDr	0.045	74
	CEM	0.047	74
10-Methyl-5-deazaacyclotetrahydrofolate	Detriot 98	2.0	74
	L	0.028	74
10-Ethyl-5-deazaacyclotetrahydrofolate	Detriot 98	0.21	74
	L	0.018	74
(6S)Dideazatetrahydrofolate	L1210	0.029	45
	CEM	0.005	48
(6R)Dideazatetrahydrofolate	L1210	0.025	45
	CEM	0.008	48
A isomer of 5-deazatetrahydrofolate	CEM	0.006	48
B isomer of 5-deazatetrahydrofolate	CEM	0.006	48

[a] These values were obtained in medium containing undialyzed fetal calf serum that probably contained some purines.

and stereoselectivity of inhibition of this enzyme by DDATHF. However, the inhibitory effect of these compounds was orders of magnitude higher against GARFT than against AICARFT. Hence, it appears that secondary effects of DDATHF against AICARFT can be uncovered by experimental conditions, such as growth of cells in AICA, but direct inhibition of AICARFT seems unlikely to be relevant to cytotoxicity or therapeutics with this compound.

Depletion of purine nucleotides. Exposure of CCRF-CEM cells to growth-inhibitory concentrations of DDATHF results in a dose-dependent diminu- ATP and GTP within 24 hours [44]. This observation is in itself instructive: It is not immediately obvious why an inhibitor of *de novo* purine synthesis would deplete ATP and GTP so dramatically when there is presumably no interference with energy metabolism. Likewise, it is not clear why DDATHF

Table 3. Relationship of antiproliferative activity, GARFT inhibition, and FPGS substrate activity for structurally-related DDATHF analogs.

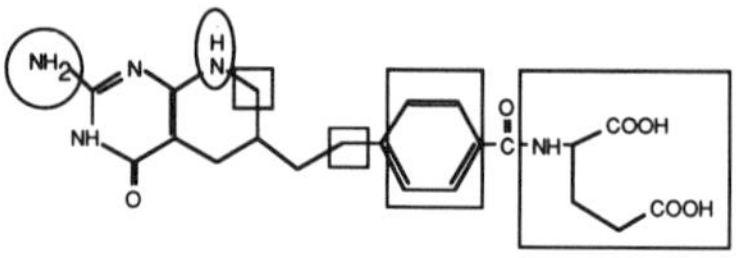

Compound	FPGS Substrate Activity	GARFT Inhibitory Activity	Tumor Cell Growth Inhibition	Ref
5,10-Dideazatetrahydrofolate	+++	++	+++	44, 45, 67
5-Deazatetrahydrofolate	++++	++	++++	48, 67
5,8,10-Trideazatetrahydrofolate	+++	-	-	71, 67
2-Desamino-5,10-dideazatetrahydrofolate	+++	-	-	67, 72
5,10-Dideazatetrahydropteroyl-L-aspartate	-	++	±	45, 67, 72
5,10-Dideazatetrahydropteroic acid	-	++	-	67, 72
5-Deazaacyclotetrahydrofolate	+++	++	++	74
5,10-Dideazaacclotetrahydrofolate	+++	++	++	67, 72, 73

The structural features of DDATHF enclosed in boxes need not be retained in order to inhibit GARFT *in vitro*, while the encircled features are essential for interaction with GARFT.

and its analogs are cytotoxic to mammalian cells, instead of simply being cytostatic. Yet, both diastereomers of DDATHF decrease the survival of mouse, hamster, and human cell lines [N. Lehrman and R.G. Moran, unpublished results].

Structure-activity relationships

The overall importance of the various biochemical processes involved in DDATHF cytotoxicity can be inferred from the patterns of antiproliferative activity of analogs of DDATHF (table 3). DDATHF differs in structure from tetrahydrofolate by substitutions of carbon for nitrogen at both positions 5 and 10. Taylor et al. [48] recently reported the synthesis and evaluation of a compound that was modified only at position 5. 5-Deazatetrahydrofolate was as active as DDATHF as an antiproliferative agent for cultured tumor cells [48] and as an inhibitor of pure GARFT [67], and was more efficiently utilized as a substrate for FPGS (figure 3B) [48]. It seems, then, that the substitution at position 5 alone was sufficient for the activity of DDATHF. Analogs of DDATHF that lacked the 2-amino group or that had an additional C for N replacement at position 8 were inactive as inhibitors of GARFT [67] and were not growth inhibitory, yet were as good substrates for FPGS as DDATHF [71]. On the other hand, 5,10-dideazatetrahydropteroyl-L-aspartate, which is not a substrate for FPGS [45], is substantially less active than DDATHF against tumor cells in culture, even with continuous exposure (figure 7B), yet is an equivalent inhibitor of isolated GARFT [67]. Likewise, 5,10-dideazatetrahydropteroic acid is as active as DDATHF against GARFT *in vitro*, yet is not a substrate for FPGS and is not cytotoxic [67,72]. The conclusions can be drawn from these correlates that antimetabolites of this class must both be inhibitory to GARFT as monoglutamates and also be metabolized to polyglutamates in order to be active cytotoxic compounds. This seems to reflect the fact that the longer chain polyglutamates of DDATHF are ~2 orders of magnitude more potent inhibitors of GARFT than DDATHF itself [67]. Interestingly, several compounds that represent moderate deviations from the structure of DDATHF, e.g., analogs in which the phenyl ring is replaced by methylene groups or the pyridine ring of DDATHF is replaced by an acyclo system (table 3), were good inhibitors of purine synthesis in intact tumor cells [73,74]. Further investigation of these compounds revealed that they both inhibited GARFT as monoglutamates and also served as substrates for FPGS [67,72,74].

Molecular modeling studies have indicated that the lowest energy conformations of (6R)DDATHF and (6S)DDATHF are remarkably similar [73]. Both molecules prefer a configuration in which the bridge region-phenyl region are at an angle of about 90° to the pyridopyrimidine ring. It was also a remarkable outcome of these calculations that the three-dimensional positions of the heterocyclic ring, the phenyl ring, and the glutamic acid of 6R and 6S diastereomers were superimposable with little or no energy cost. This would seem sufficient for an understanding of the lack of stereospecificity of the cytotoxicity of DDATHF. Thus, both FPGS [72,75] and GARFT [67] have a large tolerance for structural modifications made to the DDATHF molecule in the bridge and phenyl regions. As a result, both isomers of DDATHF can assume the same configuration and distribution in space of the heterocycle and glutamic acid regions without interfering with any binding interactions between active-site residues and the intermediate regions of the DDATHF.

Antitumor activity of DDATHF

The activity of DDTHF and the pure diastereomers of this compound that differ in chirality about carbon 6 as therapeutic agents has been extensively investigated by Dr. Gerald Grindey and his associates at Eli Lilly Research Laboratories. Summaries of Dr. Grindey's results have been published by Shih et al. [76], Beardsley et al. [77], and Taylor [78]. The parent mixture of diastereomers was originally found to be only marginally active against transplanted mouse leukemias. However, (6R,S)DDATHF was very active at preventing the growth of a spectrum of mouse solid tumors, including the antimetabolite-refractory B16 melanoma and the Lewis lung carcinoma. An exhaustive analysis of the activity of (6R)DDATHF against these tumors and against an additional battery of transplanted mouse tumors and human xenografts has demonstrated broad therapeutic activity of this compound [76].

Muggia et al. have reported the results of a phase 1 clinical trial of (6R) DDATHF [79]. The dose-limiting toxicity of the drug was myelosuppression. This effect was prolonged, delayed in onset, and cumulative in a manner very atypical of antimetabolites and more characteristic of nitrosoureas. However, myelosuppression was rapidly reversible upon administration of leucovorin (5-formyltetrahydrofolate), which proved to be a safe and effective approach to ameliorate any undue toxicity of DDATHF. A starting dose of 6 mg/m^2, given IV weekly for 3 consecutive weeks, was recommended with subsequent redosing after a 3-week interval and using leucovorin treatment for any serious myelosuppression or mucositis. During the course of this initial clinical trial, one partial response and three minor responses were noted in a population of 17 heavily pretreated patients [79]. The potency of DDATHF is extremely interesting and was not expected from the preclinical toxicology [76]; in humans, DDATHF was >1000 times more potent than 5-methyltetrahydrohomofolate [40].

Perspective

The antitumor activity of DDATHF has furnished the first evidence of the therapeutic potential of folate antimetabolites of *de novo* purine synthesis. As with any fundamentally new lead, the results obtained to date on this compound have raised more questions than they have answered. The mechanism of cell death, the reason for the large species differences in response to DDATHF, an explanation of the extreme sensitivity of human hematopoietic stem cells to this drug, and the basis for the antitumor selectivity of these agents must all be understood in order to know how these new drugs should be properly applied. However, the wealth of new insights into folate and purine metabolism and the potential for therapeutics with these compounds are powerful incentives towards the solution of these difficult questions.

Acknowledgments

This work was supported in part by grant CA27605 from the DHHS, NIH and by a Leukemia Society of America Scholar Award supported by the Scott Helping Hand Fund. I thank the investigators at Eli Lilly Research Laboratories for their supply of critical compounds and their continually collegial interactions during these studies, especially Drs. Gerald Grindey, Homer Pearce, and Joe Shih. I also acknowledge the excitement of my interactions during this work with Professors Peter Beardsley of Yale University and Ted Tayor of Princeton University, and the many surprises we have shared when dealing with these compounds. I am thankful to Angela

Bickel for her careful editorial assistance and to Dr. Franco Muggia for his critical review of the manuscript.

References

1. Jones TR, Calvert AH, Jackman AL, Brown SJ, Jones M, and Harrap KR. A potent antitumor quinazoline inhibitor of thymidylate synthetase: synthesis, biological properties, and therapeutic results in mice. Eur J Cancer 17:11–19, 1981.
2. Jackson RC, Jackman AL, and Calvert AH. Biochemical effects of a quinazoline inhibitor of thymidylate synthetase, (CB3717), on human lymphoblastoid cells. Biochem Pharmacol 32:3783–3790, 1983.
3. Moran RG, Keyomarsi K, and Patel R. Biochemical responses to treatment with fluoropyrimidines that limit tumor cell kill by these agents. In: The Expanding Role of Folates and Fluoropyrimidines in Cancer Chemotherapy, Y Rustum and JJ McGuire (eds). Plenum Press, New York, 1988, pp. 71–84.
4. Calvert AH, Alison DL, Harland SJ, Robinson BA, Jackman AL, Jones TR, Newell DR, Siddik ZH, Wiltshaw E, McElwain TJ, Smith IE, and Harrap KR. A phase I evaluation of the quinazoline antifolate thymidylate synthase inhibitor, N^{10}-propargyl-5,8-dideazafolic acid, CB3717. Clin Oncol 4:1245–1252, 1986.
5. Cantwell BMJ, Macaulay V, Harri AL, Kayl SB, Smith IE, Milsted RAV, and Calvert AH. Phase II study of the antifolate N^{10}-propargyl-5,8-deazafolic acid (CB 3717) in advanced breast cancer. Eur J Cancer Clin Oncol 24:733–736, 1988.
6. Sessa C, Zucchetti M, Ginier M, Wiellems Y, D'Incalci M, and Cavalli F. Phase I study of the antifolate N^{10}-propargyl-5,8-dideazafolic acid (CB 3717). Eur J Cancer Clin Oncol 24:769–775, 1988.
7. Patil SA, Shane B, Freisheim JH, Singh SS, and Hynes JB. Inhibition of mammalian folylpolyglutamate synthetase and human dihydrofolate reductase by 5,8-dideaza analogues of folic acid and aminopterin bearing a terminal L-ornithine. J Med Chem 32:1559–1565, 1989.
8. Cichowicz D, Cook J, George S, and Shane B. Hog liver folylpolyglutamate synthetase: substrate specificity and regulation. In: Proceeding of the Second Workshop on Folyl and Antifolyl Polyglutamates, ID Goldman (ed). Praeger Scientific, New York, 1985, pp. 7–13.
9. George S, Cichowicz DJ, and Shane B. Mammalian folylpoly-γ-glutamate synthetase. 3. Specificity for folate analogues. Biochemistry 26:522–529, 1987.
10. Rosowsky A, Freisheim JH, Moran RG, Solan VR, Bader H, Wright JE, and Radike-Smith M. Methotrexate analogues. 26. Inhibition of dihydrofolate reductase and folylpolyglutamate synthetase and *in vitro* tumor cell growth by methotrexate and aminopterin analogues containing a basic amino acid side chain. J Med Chem 29:655–660, 1986.
11. McGuire JJ, Hsieh P, Franco CT, and Piper J. Folylpolyglutamate synthetase inhibition and cytotoxic effects of methotrexate analogs containing 2, ω-diaminoalkanoic acids. Biochem Pharmacol 35:2607–2613, 1986.
12. Moran RG. Characterization of the function of mammalian folate polyglutamate synthetase. Adv Exper Med Biol 163:327–339, 1983.
13. Taylor EC, Harrington PJ, Fletcher SR, Beardsley GP, and Moran RG. Synthesis of the antileukemic agents 5,10-dideazaaminopterin and 5,10-dideaza-5,6,7,8-tetrahydroaminopterin. J Med Chem 28:914–921, 1985.
14. Moran RG, Taylor EC, and Beardsley GP. 5,10-Dideaza-5,6,7,8-tetrahydrofolate, a potent antifolate inhibitory to *de novo* purine synthesis. Proc Am Assoc Cancer Res 26:231, 1985.
15. Goodman L, DeGraw JI, Kisliuk RL, Friedkin MM, Pastore EJ, Crawford EJ, Plante LT, Nahas A, Morningstar JR, Kwok G, Wilson L, Donovan E, and Ratzan J. Tetrahydrohomofolate, a specific inhibitor of thymidylate synthetase. J Am Chem Soc 86:808–809, 1964.

16. Friedkin M, Crawford EJ, and Plante LT. Empirical vs. rational approaches in cancer chemotherapy. Ann NY Acad Sci 186:209–213, 1971.
17. Hakala MT, Zakrzewski SF, and Nichol CA. Relation of folic acid reductase to amethopterin resistance in cultured mammalian cells. J Biol Chem 236:952–958, 1961.
18. Kaufman RJ, Brown PC, and Schimke RT. Amplified dihydrofolate reductase genes in unstably methotrexate resistant cells are associated with double minute chromosomes. Proc Natl Acad Sci USA 76:5669–5673, 1979.
19. Biedler JL, Melera PW, and Spengler BA. Specifically altered metaphase chromosomes in antifolate-resistant Chinese hamster cells that overproduce dihydrofolate reductase Canc Genet Cytogenet 2:47–60, 1980.
20. Alt FW, Kellems RE, Bertino JR, and Schimke RT. Selective multiplication of dihydrofolate reductase genes in methotrexate-resistant variants of cultured murine cells. J Biol Chem 253:1357–1370, 1978.
21. Mead JAR, Goldin A. Kisliuk RL, Friedkin M, Plante L, Crawford EJ, and Kwok G. Pharmacological aspects of homofolate derivates in relation to amethopterin-resistant murine leukemia. Cancer Res 26:2374–2379, 1966.
22. Mishra LC and Mead JAR. Further evaluation of the antitumor activity of homofolate and its reduced derivatives against methotrexate-insensitive tumors. Chemotherapy 17:283–292, 1972.
23. Nichol CA and Hakala MT. Comparative growth-inhibitory activity of homofolic acid against cell lines sensitive and resistant to amethopterin. Biochem Pharmacol 15:1621–1623, 1966.
24. Diddens H, Niethammer D, and Jackson RC. Patterns of cross-resistance to the antifolate drugs trimetrexate, metoprine, homofolate, and CB 3717 in human lymphoma and osteosarcoma cells resistant to methotrexate. Cancer Res 43:5286–5292, 1983.
25. Livingston D, Crawford EJ, and Friedkin M. Studies with tetrahydrohomofolate and thymidylate synthetase in amethopterin-resistant mouse leukemia cells. Biochemistry 7: 2814–2818, 1968.
26. Thorndike J, Kisliuk RL, Gaumont Y, Piper JR, and Nair MG. Tetrahydrohomofolate polyglutamates as inhibitors of thymidylate synthase and glycinamide ribonucleotide formyltransferase in *Lactobacillius casei*. Arch Biochem Biophys 277:344–341, 1990.
27. Thorndike J, Gaumont Y, Kisliuk RL, Sirotnak FM, Murthy BR, Nair MG, and Piper JR. Inhibition of glycinamide ribonucleotide formyltransferase and other folate enzymes by homofolate polyglutamates in human lymphoma and murine leukemia cell extracts. Cancer Res 49:158–163, 1989.
28. Maley GF, Bellisario RL, Guarino DV, and Maley F. The primary sequence of *Lactobacillus casei* thymidylate synthetase. III The use of 2-(2-nitrophenylsulfenyl)-3-methyl-3-bromoindolenine and limited tryptic peptides to establish the complete amino acid sequence of the enzyme. J Biol Cem 254:1301–1304, 1979.
29. Perryman SM, Rossana C, Deng T, Vanin EF, and Johnson LF. Sequence of a complementary DNA for mouse thymidylate synthase reveals striking similarity with the prokaryotic enzymes. Mol Biol Evol 3:313–321, 1986.
30. Hakala MT. Homofolate and tetrahydrohomofolate, inhibitors of purine synthesis. Cancer Res 31:813–816, 1971.
31. Divekar AY and Hakala MT. Inhibition of the biosynthesis of 5′-phosphoribosyl-N-formylglycinamide in sarcoma 180 cells by homofolate. Mol Pharmacol 11:319–325, 1975.
32. Moran RG, Rosowsky A, and Forsch R. A new folate antimetabolite specifically inhibitory to *de novo* purine synthesis. Proc Am Assoc Cancer Res 25:311, 1984.
33. Bertrand R. and Jolivet J. Methenyltetrahydrofolate synthetase prevents the inhibition of aminoimidazole carboxamide ribonucleotide transformylase by 5-formyltetrahydrofolate polygutamates. J Biol Chem 264, 8843–8846.
34. Slieker LJ and Benkovic SJ. Inhibition of HKSV28 cell growth by 5, 11-methenyltetrahydrohomofolate. Mol Pharmacol 25:294–302, 1984.

35. Caperelli CA, Domanico P, and Benkovic SJ. Synthesis of 5, 11-methenyltetrahydrohomofolate and its antifolate activity *in vitro*. J Med Chem 24:1086–1088, 1981.
36. Forsch RA and Rosowsky A. A new one-step synthesis of leucovorin from folic acid and of 5-formyl-5,6,7,8-tetrahydrohomofolate acid from homofolic acid using dimethylamine-borane in formic acid. J Org Chem 50:2582–2583, 1985.
37. Forsch RA and Rosowsky A. A new one-step synthesis of leucovorin from folic acid and of 5-formyl-5,6,7,8-tetrahydrohomofolate acid from homofolic acid using dimethylamine-borane in formic acid. (Correction) J Org Chem 51:4326, 1986.
38. Cichowicz DJ and Shane B. Mammalian folylpoly-γ-glutamate synthetase. 2. Substrate specificity and kinetic properties. Biochemistry 26:513–521, 1987.
39. Moran RG and Colman PD. Mammalian folylpolyglutamate synthetase: partial purification and properties of the mouse liver enzyme. Biochemistry 23:4580–4589, 1984.
40. DeGraw JI, Colwell WT, Brown VH, Sato M, Kisliuk RL, Gaumont Y, Thorndike J, and Sirotnak FM. Synthesis and biological evaluation of 8-deazahomofolic acid and its tetrahydro derivative. J Med Chem 31:150–153, 1988.
41. Taylor RT and Hanna ML. 5-Methyltetrahydrohomofolate: a substrate for cobalamin methyltransferases and an inhibitor of cell growth. Arch Biochem Biophys 163:122–132, 1974.
42. Cohen GI, Parker LM, Rosowsky A, Ervin TJ, Modest EJ, and Frei E III. 5-Methyltetrahydrohomofolate (MTHTF): phase 1 trial and pharmacology in man. Proc Am Soc Clin Oncol 1:14, 1982.
43. Moran RG, Colman PD, Rosowsky A, Forsch R, and Chan KK. Structural features of 4-aminofolates requisite for substrate activity with mammalian folylpolyglutamate synthetase. Mol Pharmacol 27:156–166, 1985.
44. Beardsley GP, Taylor EC, Moroson BA, and Moran RG. 5,10-Dideaza-5,6,7,8-tetrahydrofolate, an exceptionally potent inhibitor of *de novo* purine synthesis. J Biol Chem 264:328–333, 1989.
45. Moran RG, Baldwin SW, Taylor EC, and Shih C. The 6-S and 6-R diastereomers of 5,10-dideaza-5,6,7,8-tetrahydrofolate are equiactive inhibitors of *de novo* purine synthesis. J Biol Chem 264:21047–21051, 1989.
46. Moran RG, Colman PD, and Jones TR. The relative substrate activities of structurally related pteridine, quinazoline, and pyrimidine analogs for mouse liver folylpolyglutamate synthetase. Mol Pharmacol 36:736–743, 1989.
47. Cichowicz DJ, Hynes JB, and Shane B. Substrate specificity of mammalian folylpoly-γ-glutamate synthetase for 5,8-dideazafolates and 5,8-dideaza analogues of aminopterin. Biochem Biophys Acta 957:363–369, 1988.
48. Taylor EC, Hamby JM, Shih C, Grindey GB, Rinzel SM, Beardsley GP, and Moran RG. Synthesis and antitumor activity of 5-deaza-5,6,7,8-tetrahydrofolic acid (5-DATHF) and N^{10}-substituted analogues. J Med Chem. 32:1517–1522, 1989.
49. Jackman AL, Taylor GA, O'Conner BM, Bishop JA, Moran RG, and Calvert AH. Activity of the thymidylate synthase inhibitor, 2-desamino-N10-propargyl-5,8-dideazafolic acid and related compounds in murine (L1210) and human (W1L2) systems *in vitro* and *in vivo*. Cancer Res 50:5212–5218, 1990.
50. Henderson JF. Feedback inhibition of purine biosynthesis in ascites tumor cells. J Biol Chem 237:2631–2635, 1962.
51. DeGraw JI, Christie PH, Kisliuk RL, Gaumont Y, and Sirotnak FM. Synthesis and antifolate properties of 10-alkyl-5,10-dideaza analogues of methotrexate and tetrahydrofolic acid. J Med Chem 33:673–677, 1990.
52. Barnett C and Wilson TM. Asymmetric synthesis and absolute configuration of 5,10-dideaza-5,6,7,8-tetrahydropteroic acid and 5,10-dideaza-5,6,7,8-tetrahydrofolic acid (DDATHF). In: Chemistry and Biology of Pteridines, 1989. Pteridine and Folic Acid Derivatives, H Ch Curtis, S Ghisla, and N Blau (eds). De Gruyter Publishing, New York, 1990, pp. 102–105.

53. Dev IK and Harvey RJ. N10-formyltetrahydrofolate is the formyl donor for gylcinamide ribonucleotide transformylase in *Escherichia cali*. J Biol Chem 253:4242–4244, 1978.
54. Smith GK, Benkovic PA, and Benkovic SJ. L(-)-10-formyltetrahydrofolate is the cofactor for glycinamide ribonucleotide transformylase from chicken liver. Biochemistry 20:4034–4036, 1981.
55. McGuire JJ, Hsieh P, Coward JJ, and Bertino JR. Enzymatic synthesis of folylpolyglutamates: characterization of the reaction and its products. J Biol Chem 255: 5776–5788, 1980.
56. Sato JK and Moran RG. Interaction of methotrexate and citrovorum factor with folylpolyglutamate synthetase. Proc Am Assoc Cancer Res 25:312, 1984.
57. Boschelli DH, Webber S, Whitely JM, Oronsky AL, and Kerwar SS. Synthesis and biological properties of 5,10-dideaza-5,6,7,8-tetrahydrofolic acid. Arch Biochem Biophys 265:43–49, 1988.
58. Sirotnak FM, Otter G, Piper JR, and DeGraw JI. Analogs of tetrahydrofolate directed at folate-dependent purine biosynthetic enzymes. Characteristics of mediated entry and transport-related resistance in L1210 cells for 5,10-dideazatetrahydrofolate and two alkyl derivatives. Biochem Pharmacol 37:4775–4777, 1990.
59. Beardsley GP, Taylor EC, Shih C, Poore GA, Grindey GB, and Moran RG. A new class of antifolates, 5,10-dideazatetrahydrofolic acid, an inhibitor of GAR transformylase with broad *in vivo* activity. Proc Am Assoc Cancer Res 27:259, 1986.
60. Pizzorno G, Russello O, Cashmore AR, Moroson BA, Cross AD, Coronnello M, and Beardsley GP. Polyglutamation: an essential step in the activation of 5,10-dideazatetrahydrofolic acid. Proc Am Assoc Cancer Res 31:339, 1990.
61. Fry DW, Anderson LA, Borst M, and Goldman ID. Analysis of the role of methotrexate in gut and the Ehrlich tumor *in vivo* as factors in drug sensitivity and selectivity. Cancer Res 43:1087–1092, 1983.
62. Galivan J. Evidence for the cytotoxic activity of polyglutamate derivatives of methotrexate. Mol Pharmacol 17:105–110, 1980.
63. Sikora E, Jackman AL, Newell DR, and Calver AH. Formation, retention, and biological activity of N^{10} propargyl-5,8-deazafolic acid (CB 3717) polyglutamates in L1210 cells *in vitro*. Biochem Pharmacol 37:4047–4054, 1988.
64. Pizzorno G, Cashmore AR, Moroson BA, and Beardsley GP. Leucovorin (LV): a 'rescue' agent for 5,10-dideazatetrahydrofolic acid (DDATHF). Proc Am Assoc Cancer Res 31:339, 1990.
65. Pizzorno G, Cashmore AR, Moroson BA, Cross AR, Shih C, and Beardsley GP. Enhanced target enzyme levels, impaired polyglutamation, and enhanced pools of natural folates are associated with resistance to deazatetrahydrofolates in CCRF-CEM cells. Proc Am Assoc Cancer Res 30:480, 1989.
66. Galivan J, Nimec Z, Boschelli D, Oronsky AL, and Kerwar SS. Antifolate drug interactions: enhancement of growth inhibition due to the antipurine 5,10-dideazatetrahydrofolic acid by the lipophilic dihydrofolate reductase inhibitors metoprine and trimetrexate. Cancer Res 48:2421–2425, 1988.
67. Baldwin SW, Tse A, Taylor EC, Rosowsky A, Shih C, and Moran RG. Structural features of 5,10-dideaza-5,6,7,8-tetrahydrofolate that determine inhibition of mammalian glycinamide ribonucleotide formyltransferase. Biochemistry 30:1997–2006, 1991.
68. Jackson RC, Hart LI, and Harrap KR. Intrinsic resistance to methotrexate of cultured mammalian cells in relation to the inhibition kinetics of their dihydrofolate reductases. Cancer Res 36:1991–1997, 1976.
69. Strauss OH and Goldstein A. Zone behavior of enzymes. J Gen Physiol 26:559–585, 1943.
70. Werkheiser WC. Specific binding of 4-aminofolic acid analogues by folic acid reductase. J Biol Chem 236:888–893, 1961.
71. Rosowsky A, Forsch RA, and Moran RG. 5,8,10-Trideaza-5,6,7,8-tetrahydropteroyl-L-glutamate and -L-ornithine as potential antifolates and antitumor agents. J Med Chem 32:709–715, 1989.

72. Moran RG, Colman PD, Taylor EC, and Shih C. Polyglutamation determines the antitumor activity of deazatetrahydrofolate inhibitors of purine synthesis. Cancer Res, submitted, 1991.
73. Shih C, Grindey GB, Moran RG, and Taylor EC. Molecular modelling studies on deazatetrahydrofolates. In: Chemistry and Biology of Pteridines, 1989. Pteridine and Folic Acid Derivatives, H Ch Curtis, S Ghisla, and N Blau (eds). De Gruyter Publishing, New York, 1990, pp. 995–1000.
74. Kelly JL, McLean EW, Cohn NK, Edelstein MP, Duch DS, Smith GK, Hanlon MH, and Ferone R. Synthesis and biological activity of an acyclic analogue of 5,6,7,8-tetrahydrofolic acid, N-[4-[[3-(2,4-diamino-1,6-dihydro-6-oxo-5-pyrimidinyl)propyl]amino]-benzoyl]-L-glutamic acid. J Med Chem 33:561–567, 1990.
75. Moran RG, Shih C, Taylor EC, and Rosowsky A. Acylic folates analogs retain activity as substrates for mouse liver folylpolyglutamate synthetase (FPGS). Proc Am Assoc Cancer Res. 30:478, 1989.
76. Shih C, Grindey GB, Houghton PJ, and Houghton J. *In vivo* antitumor activity of 5,10-dideazatetrahydrofolic acid (DDATHF) and its diastereomeric isomers. Proc Am Assoc Cancer Res 29:283, 1988.
77. Beardsley GP, Taylor EC, Grindey GB, and Moran RG. Deaza derivatives of tetrahydrofolic acid. A new class of folate antimetabolites. In: Chemistry and Biology of the Pteridines, 1986. BA Cooper and VM Whitehead (eds). De Gruyter and Co., New York, 1986, pp. 953–957.
78. Taylor EC. New pathways from pteridines. Design and synthesis of a new class of potent and selective antitumor agents. J Heter Chem 27:1–12, 1990.
79. Muggia F, Martin T, Ray M, Leichman CG, Grunberg S, Gill I, Moran R, Dyke R, and Grindey G. Phase 1 clinical trial of weekly 5,10-dideazatetrahydrofolate (LY 26418, DDATHF-B) Proc Am Assoc Clin Oncol 9:74, 1990.

5. Taxol: A new agent active in melanoma and ovarian cancer

Avi I. Einzig, Peter H. Wiernik, and Edward L. Schwartz

Introduction

Taxol was isolated in 1971 from the stem bark of the plant *Taxus brevifolia*, (western yew), a small evergreen native to the Pacific Northwest, and its structure was characterized by Wani et al. [1]. This drug is a complex ester, consisting of a taxane derivative with an oxetan ring, an unusual chemical structure (as shown in figure 1) whose biological activity had not been previously studied.

Taxol is a potent inhibitor of cell replication that blocks cells in the late G_2 or M phases of the cell cycle [2]. As seen by immunofluorescence with tubulin antibodies and electron microscopy, taxol-treated cells exhibit an unusual microtuble cytoskeleton. In addition to their cytoplasmic microtubules, they display prominent bundles of microtubules. Incubation of cells with taxol results in the stabilization of cellular microtubules to depolymerization by cold [2, 3]. The presence of bundles of microtubules is characteristic of the cytoskeleton of taxol-treated cells and has been reported in a number of cell lines [2, 4–9].

The inhibition of HeLa and BALB/C fibroblast cell replication in the presence of low concentrations of taxol could derive from the cell being unable to depolymerize its cytoskeleton. This may help explain the mechanism of action and partially account for the observed antitumor activity of taxol. Little is known about the biological machinery involved in cell migration. The microtubule cytoskeleton may play a role by determining the polarity of migrating cells. Experiments suggest that migrating cells must be able to both polymerize and depolymerize their cytoplasmic microtubules in order to migrate [2].

In contrast with other antimitotic agents that inhibit microtubule polymerization in vitro, taxol enhances both the rate and yield of microtubule assembly by shifting the equilibrium between the tubulin dimer and polymer in favor of the polymer [10]. Though experiments done with taxol in vitro indicate that more tubulin is in the form of polymer, the microtubules are shorter than those seen in its absence, suggesting that taxol is responsible for

Franco M. Muggia (ed.), NEW DRUGS, CONCEPTS AND RESULTS IN CANCER CHEMOTHERAPY.

Kluwer Academic Publishers, Boston. *ISBN 0-7923-1253-8*

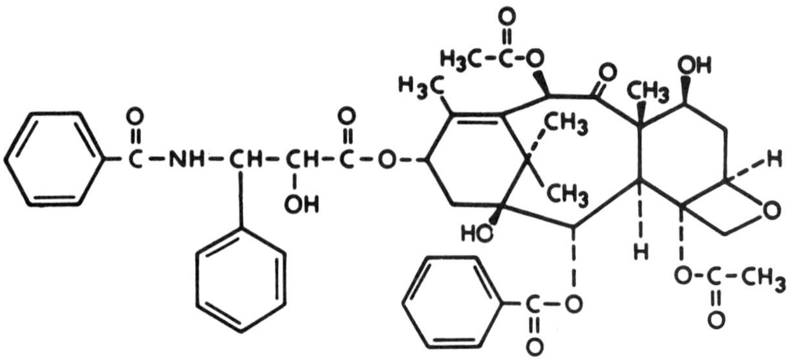

TAXOL

Figure 1.

increasing the number of nucleation events at the start of microtubule assembly [11].

The drug has a unique capacity to assemble tubulin into its polymer form. The critical concentration of microtubule protein required for assembly is reduced in the presence of taxol, and the microtubules formed are stable to depolymerization by calcium or cold. Taxol also assembles tubulin under conditions in which polymerization would not normally occur.

Evidence suggests that there is a taxol binding site on the microtubule. This binding site is distinct from the binding sites for colchicine, podophyllotoxin, or vinblastine [12, 13].

The enhancement of both the rate and yield of microtubule assembly and the presence of a binding site on the polymer makes taxol distinct from all other antimitotic agents whose mechanism of action have been analyzed. The drug exhibits specificity for the tubulin-microtubule system. Taxol does not influence actin polymerization or bind to intermediate filaments or DNA [14].

Although taxol was found to demonstrate moderate activity against the L1210 lymphoid leukemia in 1967, it was not selected for development to clinical trial until 1977. At that time, the selection was based on its activity against the murine B16 melanoma. It subsequently demonstrated good activity against the human MX-1 mammary tumor xenograft and moderate activity against both the intraperitoneally implanted L1210 and P388 leukemias, and also against the CX-1 colon and LX-1 lung xenografts. Taxol was not effective against the murine CD8F, mammary and colon 38 carcinomas, and the implanted Lewis lung carcinoma [15].

Preclinical toxicology

Preclinical toxicology studies were done with taxol by intraperitoneal administration in Sprague-Dawley rats and CD2F1 mice, and by intravenous infusion in beagle dogs. The rat and dog studies were done on either a single dose or a five consecutive daily dose schedule, while the mouse toxicity study was done on the daily × 5 schedule only.

Female mice were slightly less sensitive to taxol then males; based upon a comparison of LD_{50} and LD_{10} values, both sexes had an equivalent response at the LD_{90} in all cases.

The intraperitoneal route was selected as the closest approximation to the intravenous route, which was precluded in rodent studies due to dose volume constraints imposed by limited compound solubility and vehicle toxicity. Rapid intravascular absorption from the peritoneal cavity was anticipated due to the lipophilic nature of taxol, and observed toxicity evidenced that absorption had occurred. The intravenous infusion (2.0 ml/min) was used in the beagle dog studies.

Dose-related reversible myelosuppression, characterized by suppression of both lymphocytes and neutrophils, was the major toxicity attributable to taxol in both rats and dogs. Dose-related, reversible, lymphoid depletion of the thymus was observed in mice. Evidence of erythroid toxicity in rodents was limited to reversible, dose-related decreases in circulating reticulocytes in both species, and dogs were more affected than rodents. Thrombocytopenia was observed in dogs and in rats. No effects on the reproductive system were noted in the female of any species, or in male dogs.

No histologic evidence of cardiac toxicity was found in these studies. However, clinical observations suggested a cardiovascular effect, probably related to the vehicle. Acute deaths were observed within ½ to 1 hour after dosing, and clinical signs, including vasodilation, hypothermia, labored or difficult breathing, and lethargy, were observed in these dogs prior to death and were compatible with hypotensive shock. Dogs have been previously reported to be sensitive to the hypotensive effects of cremophor, the vehicle in which taxol is administered.

No histological evidence of drug or vehicle-related toxicity to the central or peripheral nervous system was seen in any species. However, clinical signs suggestive of central nervous system effects were noted. Pronounced lethargy and difficulty in breathing were seen in high volume in dogs, which may have been related to the hypotensive effects of the cremophor vehicle component.

Aside from sporadic, reversible incidences of increased BUN, no evidence of any renal effects was noted, and there was no histological evidence of liver toxicity.

The LD_{10} of taxol in mice on a daily × 5-day schedule was 70 mg/m^2/day. In the dog studies, the highest nontoxic dose of taxol was 22.5 mg/m^2 with the single dose and 7.5 mg/m^2 on the daily × 5-day schedule. The respective figures for the toxic low dose (TDL) were 45 mg/m^2 on the single dose and 15 mg/m^2/day for 5 days on the divided-dose schedule.

Clinical pharmacokinetics

Three of the phase I clinical trials yielded detailed pharmacokinetic information [16–18]. Data from the 6-hour IV infusion trial showed that taxol disappearance from plasma was biphasic; half-lives of the first and second phases after a 275 mg/m^2 dose were 0.32 and 8.6 hours, respectively. The apparent volume of distribution was 95 l/m^2, and the peak plasma concentration with a dose of 275 mg/m^2, which occurred immediately postinfusion, was approximately 8 μM. Only 5% of parent drug was excreted in the urine within 24 hours. When taxol was administered as a 1-hour or 6-hour IV infusion, the plasma disappearance was best characterized as a bioexponential process. Despite extensive protein binding, the drug appeared to be readily eliminated from plasma. Urinary clearance was rather insignificant and suggested that metabolism, biliary excretion, and/or extensive tissue binding are responsible for the bulk of systemic drug clearance. When taxol was administered as a 24-hour infusion, plasma concentrations increased during the 24-hour infusion period and began to decline immediately upon cessation of drug infusion.

Phase I clinical trials

Phase I studies were initiated using various schedules. Because of the concern for the hypotensive effects of the cremophor vehicle, the initial trials were limited to the 5-day divided-dose schedule. Between May and December 1984, Legha et al. [19] at M.D. Anderson Hospital conducted a phase I study of taxol using a 5-day intermittent schedule. Twenty patients with metastatic solid tumors refractory to standard therapy were entered. The dose of taxol ranged from 5 to 40 mg/m^2 daily for 5 days and was repeated at 3-week intervals. The daily dosage of taxol was infused over a period of 1 hour. Nausea and vomiting were uncommon and required no antiemetic therapy. A mild to moderate degree of diarrhea was observed in six patients. Mild stomatitis was experienced by two patients at the higher dose levels. Alopecia was a prominent side effect, occurring in nearly every patient treated in the dose range of 30–40 mg/m^2. No acute hypersensitivity reactions were observed. The dose-limiting toxicity of taxol in this study was myelosuppression, which was expressed predominantly as leukopenia. At the dose level of 30 mg/m^2, neutropenia developed in all patients. Taxol therapy had a very minimal effect on platelet counts, with the majority of patients maintaining normal platelet counts. The myelosuppressive toxicity of taxol was generally predictable, noncumulative, and reversible. Among the 20 patients treated with taxol, 18 were evaluable for response and no objective regression of tumor was observed. Using the 5-day schedule of drug administration, their data supported a starting taxol dose of 30 mg/m^2 daily for phase II trials.

The phase I trial of taxol at the Johns Hopkins Oncology Center [20] utilized a single infusion schedule every 21 days. Thirty patients were enrolled in the study and dosages were escalated from 15 to 265 mg/m^2. The infusions were initially given over 1 hour. A major concern in the initiation of the study was the possibility of acute cardiopulmonary toxicity or hypersensitivity reactions. Between the doses of 15 and 135 mg/m^2, when the drug was given over 1 hour, five such reactions of varying severity were observed. These data, along with those from other centers reporting a similarly high rate of acute reactions, prompted a change in the schedule of administration. Since 2 of the 5 acute episodes occurred during the first course of treatment, there was no indication that prior exposure was a risk for toxicity. The pathophysiology of these reactions could not be ascertained. It was decided to proceed with the trial with a schedule of premedication modeled after that described for patients with a severe previous reaction to IV radiocontrast medium [21]. The duration of infusion was also prolonged to a 6-hour infusion in which the rate of infusion was started slowly and increased over the initial 2 hours. The final 14 patients received taxol on this schedule, with three reactions, only one of which required discontinuation of the drug. Nausea and vomiting were mild and infrequently seen, as were mucositis and diarrhea. Symptomatic sensory neuropathy was a common finding at the three highest doses. Myelosuppression, principally leukopenia, was the dose-limiting toxicity in this study, and thrombocytopenia occurred infrequently. Alopecia was universal. The leukopenia was clearly dose related, with nadirs occurring between days 8 and 13, with prompt recovery. Based on their data, they recommended doses of 170 and 212 mg/m^2 for heavily and minimally previously treated patients, respectively, for phase II studies. There was evidence of antitumor effect in two patients. One patient with an adenocarcinoma of the lung had a decrease in CEA, and a second patient with epithelial ovarian cancer had a decrease in multiple measurable peritoneal masses on CT scan and a disappearance of gross ascites for 5 months.

Taxol was administered to 34 patients in an initial phase I study at Albert Einstein Cancer Center [16]. An acute hypersensitivity reaction occurred in 3 of the first 4 patients treated. This trial utilized an IV infusion over 6 hours every 3 weeks, with a starting dose of 15 mg/m^2. A premedication regimen of dexamethasone, diphenhydramine, and cimetidine was instituted after the initial reactions, and no further reactions occurred. Hematological toxicity manifested as leukopenia and neutropenia at doses of 175 mg/m^2 and greater was observed. Platelet counts and hematocrit were not affected by the treatment. The grade of leukopenia was variable at all doses (175 mg/m^2 and greater) and among courses of treatment for each patient.

Neurotoxicity was dose limiting at 275 mg/m^2. The neuropathy was described as predominantly sensory, often associated with pain. Quantitative sensory testing revealed significant elevations in vibration thresholds in five patients and thermal threshold elevations in two patients. Nerve conduction velocities in one patient showed slowing in sensory nerves, with relative sparing of motor nerves. Sensory symptoms resolved several months after treatment was discontinued.

Two colon cancer patients who had progressive disease prior to taxol had stable disease after treatment. One patient who was treated with five courses of taxol underwent laporatomy in preparation for intraperitoneal chemotherapy and had significant tumor necrosis; the other patient had stable disease for 4.5 months with a 50% decrease in plasma CEA. Complete disappearance of skin lesions occurred for month in a patient with gastric carcinoma. A minor response in an abdominal mass and a partial reduction of a pulmonary nodule lasting 6 weeks was noted in a patient with ovarian cancer. A partial response with complete resolution of massive ascites lasting 6 months occurred in a male patient with adenocarcinoma of unknown origin. These objective responses suggested that taxol had activity against adenocarcinoma, and the recommended phase II dose with this schedule was 250 mg/m^2.

A 24-hour continuous intravenous infusion schedule was adopted in another phase I study at Albert Einstein Cancer Center [17]. Twenty-six patients were treated in this study with taxol and the premedicaton regimen described above. The starting dose was 150 mg/m^2, and escalation to 275 mg/m^2 was possible. Peripheral neuropathy was determined to be the dose-limiting toxicity. Neuropathy was initially observed at 200 mg/m^2 and increased in severity at 250 mg/m^2 and 275 mg/m^2. Bone marrow suppression, primarily manifested as neutropenia, was observed at all doses tested, with no significant difference in the grade of myelosuppression with increasing dosage. One patient developed stridor during her second course of therapy and was treated for presumed acute hypersensitivity.

Taxol was shown to have activity in metastatic melanoma in this study, with 4 of 12 patients achieving a partial response. These responses were observed in skin lesions, lymph nodes, and soft-tissue masses. This study suggested that taxol can be safely administered to patients with premedication to avoid acute hypersensitivity reactions and that 250 mg/m^2 was an appropriate phase II dose on this schedule. Furthermore, the study demonstrated that taxol has significant activity against melanoma.

Sixteen patients were entered in a phase I trial at the University of Wisconsin Clinical Cancer Center [22] utilizing a short IV infusion daily for 5 days in patients with refractory solid tumors. The starting dose was 5 mg/m^2/day and was escalated to 40 mg/m^2/day. The initial patients received taxol over 60 minutes but 2 of the first 5 patients treated developed anaphylactoid reactions during the infusion. Patients were subsequently premedicated with prednisone, diphenhydramine, and cimetidine, and the infusion was extended to 6 hours.

Myelosuppression was dose limiting at 40 mg/m^2/day × 5. Other toxicities included mild to moderate nausea and vomiting in a minority of patients, and moderate alopecia in one patient. Neurologic toxicity was not observed. No complete or partial responses were observed.

A phase I trial of taxol was administered as a 3-hour IV infusion every 21 days at Memorial Sloan Kettering Cancer Center to 28 patients with escalating doses from 15 to 230 mg/m^2 [23]. Hypersensitivity reactions characterized by acute dyspnea and erythema occurred in three patients, with one episode leading to irreversible hypotension and death. Patients were not premedicated in that study. Leukopenia was observed, as well as thrombocytopenia, mild to moderate nausea or emesis, stomatitis, and alopecia. Hypersensitivity reactions were a treatment-limiting toxicity of taxol given on this schedule without premedication.

Another phase I study at Mt. Sinai Hospital in New York [24] administered taxol as a 24-hour intravenous infusion. The dose-limiting toxicity was leukopenia at 200 mg/m^2. No anaphylactic reactions occurred in this study without premedication. One patient with colon carcinoma had a transient decrease in tumor mass, and a patient with head and neck carcinoma had a decrease in the size of a neck nodule.

Initial phase I trials resulted in a significant incidence of acute hypersensitivity reactions, which were assumed to be caused by the cremophor vehicle and were infusion-rate related. As a result, routine premedication was recommended with cimetidine, dexamethasone, and diphenhydramine in subsequent trials. Koeller et al. [25] conducted a phase I trial in which taxol was administered as a 6-hour infusion every 21 days without premedication. Thirty patients were treated, with only one patient experiencing a hypersensitivity reaction, and that patient was safely retreated with premedication. Dose-limiting toxicity was myelosuppression at 275 mg/m^2. There were two partial responses (squamous cell carcinoma of the lung, adenocarcinoma of unknown primary). Based on these data, the role of premedication in preventing an acute hypersensitivity reaction is questionable. Further elucidation of the hypersensitivity reaction is necessary before a conclusion can be reached regarding the role of premedication in preventing it.

A phase I study of taxol in leukemia has been conducted by Rowinsky et al. at Johns Hopkins Hospital [26]. Taxol was administered as a 24-hour continuous infusion with a starting dose of 200 mg/m^2, which was escalated to 390 mg/m^2. Mucositis was the dose-limiting toxicity in this study. The severity of neurosensory toxicity was dose related, with moderate paresthesias and sensory loss at the 315 mg/m^2 and 390 mg/m^2 levels. Myelosuppression was consistently observed at all dose levels, but there were no complete responses, and only one partial response was observed in a patient with acute lymphocytic leukemia.

Phase II clinical trials

Phase II studies of taxol in metastatic melanoma [27–28], renal-cell carcinoma [29], and ovarian cancer [30, 31, 31A] have been published.

A phase II study of taxol at Albert Einstein Cancer Center administered as a 24-hour continuous intravenous infusion at 275 mg/m^2 in patients with metastatic melanoma demonstrated three complete responses (11 weeks, 25+ months, 38+ months) and a partial response of 5 months duration among 28 evaluable patients. Responses were observed in nodal and soft-tissue lesions. Toxicities included myelosuppression, alopecia, and peripheral neuropathy. Premedication with dexamethasone, diphenhydramine, and cimetidine was utilized, and there were four episodes of acute hypersensitivity reactions. A phase II study at MD Anderson achieved 3 partial responses out of 25 evaluable patients [28].

Another phase II study of taxol at the Albert Einstein Cancer Center administered as a continuous intravenous infusion at 275 mg/m^2 in 18 evaluable patients with metastatic renal-cell carcinoma resulted in no objective responses.

In a phase II study at Johns Hopkins Hospital conducted by McGuire et al. [30] in advanced ovarian cancer, taxol was administered as a 24-hour, continuous intravenous infusion at a starting dose of 170 or 135 mg/m^2 for minimally or heavily pretreated patients, respectively. Forty patients are evaluable for response with 1 pathologic complete response, 11 clinical partial responses, and 6 clinical minor responses. The complete response continues for 8+ months, and the partial responses have ranged from 66 to 363+ days. Dose-limiting toxicity was neutropenia.

A phase II study at the Albert Einstein Cancer Center was conducted by Einzig et al. [31] in advanced ovarian cancer with taxol administered as a 24-hour continuous intravenous at a starting dose of 250 mg/m^2, with dose deescalation for severe neutropenia, thrombocytopenia, or peripheral neuropathy. One complete and five partial responses were documented out of 30 evaluable patients.

The Gynecologic Oncology Group also conducted a phase II study of taxol in ovarian cancer as a 24 hr continuous infusion at a dose of 175 mg/m^2. Five complete and 10 partial responses were reported [31A].

Future trials

There is continuing interest in taxol by clinical researchers, although the progress has been hampered by an inadequate supply of the drug. In 1987 the National Cancer Institute ordered 60,000 pounds of the bark from forests in California, Oregon, and Washington so that clinical trials of taxol can proceed. Although chemists are making progress in the synthesis of taxol [32], it is a complex molecule that is difficult to prepare in the laboratory.

The formulation of taxol for clinical trials could be improved if extreme insolubility in aqueous solvents could be overcome. The current vehicle, cremophor, has been implicated as the cause of the hypersensitivity reactions, which has been observed in most trials. In an attempt to improve the solubility characteristics of the drug, information about the chemical structure of the drug as it relates to biological activity has been sought. A number of natural and semisynthetic congeners of taxol have been studied [33]. Experiments have indicated that both an intact taxane ring and an ester side chain at position C-13 are required for cytotoxicity in cells growing in tissue culture.

Information on the effects of chemical alterations of the taxol molecule on biological activity will increase our knowledge concerning the interaction of the drug with its cellular target, the regulation of microtubule assembly, and the identification of mitosis-specific microtubule-associated proteins.

In addition to antitumor activity, taxol may be helpful as a tumor-cell synchronizing agent. The usefulness of taxol as a cell synchronizing agent depends on the drug's ability to block cells in metaphase and the cell's ability to reverse this block. The tumor cells would need to proceed through the cell cycle maintaining their synchrony and be susceptible to drugs that inhibit DNA synthesis as they enter the S phase of the cell cycle [34].

Taxol has activity in melanoma and ovarian cancer. Phase III studies with taxol are indicated in these diseases. Additional phase II clinical trials should be conducted in other solid tumors. Other methods of administration, including intraperitoneally, and the combination of taxol with other active agents may increase its efficacy and combination with G-CSF may decrease its toxicity.

Neurotoxic neuropathy

Dose-limiting neurotoxicity has been observed in 2 of the 7 phase I trials of taxol. Tissue culture studies provide a potential mechanism for the observed neurotoxicity [35–40]. In organotypic dorsal root ganglion spinal-cord cultures, taxol exposure leads to the formation of unusual numbers and arrays of microtubules in neurons, satellite cells, and Schwann cells [41–43]. In vivo, the dorsal root ganglion cells are particularly vulnerable to neurotoxins because of the special permeability of their blood vessels. The predominance of sensory features in the clinically observed neuropathy and the rapid onset with early symptoms in the hands and feet suggest that this is a neuropathy affecting the sensory ganglia or myelin sheath [44]. Electrophysiologic data [45] support the presence of both axonal degeneration and demyelination. In the clinical trials, treatment discontinuation or deescalation of dosage was necessary because of neurotoxicity. A mechanism for diminishing neurotoxicity might permit the administration of higher doses of taxol. It has been shown [44,46] that nerve growth factor (NGF), a neuronotrophic factor normally required for maintenance of sympathetic and dorsal root ganglion (DRG) neurons in tissue culture, attenuates the cytotoxic effects of taxol in DRG explant cultures. The gene for human NGF has been cloned; it is possible that administration of a neuronotrophic factor, along with taxol, may limit the neurotoxicity and extend the useful dosage range of the drug.

Taxol-resistant cells

A drug-resistant cell line was developed over a 1-year period by growing J774.2 cells in the presence of stepwise increases in the concentration of taxol [47]. The taxol-resistant cell line demonstrated a major reduction in steady-state accumulation of taxol compared with the parental cell line. The plasma membranes of the resistant cells included a phosphoglycoprotein with an approximate molecular weight of 135 kDa that was essentially not detected in the taxol-sensitive cells. The presence of the 135-kDa phosphoglycoprotein in the plasma membranes of taxol-resistant cells correlated well with resistance to the drug. Resistance to the growth-inhibitory properties of taxol was extremely dependent on the presence of the drug [48]. Analysis of tubulin from these resistant cells did not indicate any major alterations as compared with tubulin in the drug-sensitive cells. This taxol-resistant cell line is related to a category of drug-resistant cells that has been described as multidrug resistant [49]. Such cells have a distinctive phenotype, which includes cross-resistance to drugs that are structurally unrelated; altered permeability properties, which result in a reduced intracellular accumulation of drug; and the presence of a high molecular weight glycoprotein in their plasma membranes. There are often alterations in karyotype, such as the inclusion of double-minute chromosomes and homogeneously staining regions that indicate gene amplification. Although the function of the membrane glycoprotein is not completely understood, it has been proposed to function as an efflux pump that maintains the amount of antitumor drug within the cell below the cytotoxic level [50–52].

References

1. Wani MC, Taylor HL, Wall ME, et al. Plant antitumor agents. VI. The isolation and structure of taxol, a novel antileukemic and antitumor agent from *Taxus brevifolia*. Am Chem Soc 93:2325–2327, 1971.
2. Schiff PB and Horwitz SB. Taxol stabilizes microtubules in mouse fibroblast cells. Proc Natl Acad Sci USA 77:1561–1565, 1980.
3. Crossin KL and Carney DH. Microtubule stabilization by taxol inhibits initiation of DNA synthesis by thrombin and by epidermal growth factor. Cell 27:341–350, 1981.
4. DeBrabander M, Gruens G, Nuydens R, et al. Taxol induces the assembly of free microtubules in living cells and blocks the organizing capacity of the centrosomes and kineto-

chores. Proc Natl Acad Sci USA 78:5608–5612, 1981.
5. DeBrabander M. A model for the microtubule organizing activity of the centrosomes and kinetochores in mammalion cells. Cell Biol Int Rep 6:901–915, 1982.
6. Albertini DF and Clark JI. Visualization of assembled and disassembled microtubule protein by double label fluorescence microscopy. Cell Biol Int Rep 5:387–397, 1981.
7. Brenner SL and Brinkley BB. Tubulin assembly sites and the organization of microtubule arrays in mammalion cells. Cold Spring Harbor Symp Quant Biol. 46:241–254, 1982.
8. Tokunaka S, Friedman TM, Toyama Y, et al. Taxol induces microtubule-rough endoplasmic reticulum complexes and microtubule-bundles in cultured chondroblasts. Differentiation 24:39–47, 1983.
9. Manfredi JJ, Parness J, and Horwitz SB, Taxol binds to cellular microtubules. J Cell Biol 94:688–696, 1982.
10. Schiff PB, Fant J, and Horwitz SB. Promotion of nicrotubule assembly in vitro by taxol. Nature (London) 277:665–667, 1979.
11. Schiff PB and Horwitz SB: Tubulin: A target for chemotherapeutic agents. In: Molecular Actions and Targets for Cancer Chemotherapeutic Agents, Vol. 2, AC Sartorelli, JS Lazo, JR Bertino (eds). Bristol-Myers Cancer Symposium. Academic Press, New York, 1981, pp. 483–507.
12. Schiff PB and Horwitz SB: Taxol assembles tubulin in the absence of exogenous 5′-triphosphate or microtubule-associated proteins. Biochemistry 20:3247–3252, 1981.
13. Kumar N. Taxol-induced polymerization of purified tubulin. J Biol Chem 256:10435–10441, 1981.
14. Parness J and Horwitz SB. Taxol binds to polymerized tubulin in vitro. J Cell Biol 91:479–487, 1981.
15. National Cancer Institute Clinical Brochure. Taxol (NSC 125973), 1990.
16. Wiernik PH, Schwartz EL, Strauman JJ, et al. Phase I clinical and pharmacokinetic study of taxol. Cancer Res. 47:2486–2493, 1987.
17. Wiernik PH, Schwartz EL, Einzig A, et al. Phase I trial of taxol given as a 24-hour infusion every 21 days: Responses observed in metastatic melanoma. J Clin Oncol 5:1232–1239, 1987.
18. Longnecker SW, Donehower RC, Cates AE, et al. High performance liquid chromatographic assay for taxol in human plasma and urine and pharmacokinetics in a phase I trial. Cancer Treat Rep 71:53–59, 1987.
19. Legha SS, Tenney DM, and Krakoff IR. Phase I study of taxol using a 5-day intermittent schedule. J Clin Oncol 4:762–766, 1986.
20. Donehower RC, Rowinsky EK, Grochow LB, et al. Phase I trial of taxol in patients with advanced cancer. Cancer Treat Rep. 71:1171–1177, 1987.
21. Greenberger PA, Patterson R, Simon R, et al. Pretreatment of high risk patients requiring radiographic contrast media studies. J Allergy Clin Immunol 67:185–187, 1981.
22. Grem JL, Kendro DT, Simon KJ, et al. Phase I study of taxol administered as a short IV infusion daily for 5 days. Cancer Treat Rep 71:1179–1184, 1987.
23. Kris MG, O'Connell JP, Gralla RJ. et al. Phase I trial of taxol given as a 3-hour infusion every 21 days. Cancer Treat Rep 70:605–607, 1986.
24. Ohnuma T, Zimet AS, Coffey VA, et al. Phase I study of taxol in a 24-hr. infusion schedule. Proc Ann Meet Am Assoc Cancer Res 26:167, 1985.
25. Koeller J, Brown T, Havlin K, et al. A phase I/pharmacokinetic study of taxol given by a prolonged infusion without premedication. Proc Ann Meet Am Soc Clin Oncol 8:82, 1989.
26. Rowinsky EK, Donehower RC, Jones RJ, et al. Microtubule changes and cytotoxicity in leukemic cell lines treated with taxol. Cancer Res 48:4093–4100, 1988.
27. Einzig AI, Hochster H, Wiernik PH, et al. A phase II study of taxol in patients with malignant melanoma. Invest New Drugs 9:59–64, 1991.
28. Legha SS, Ring S, Papadopoulus N, et al. Taxol: a phase II study in patients with malignant melanoma. Cancer 65:2478–2481, 1990.
29. Einzig AI, Gorowski E, Sasloff J, et al. Phase II trial of taxol in patients with metastatic renal cell carcinoma. Cancer Invest 9:133–136, 1991.

30. McGuire WP, Rowinsky EK, Rosenshein NB, et al. Taxol: a unique antineoplastic agent with significant activity in advanced ovarian epithelial neoplasms. Ann Intern Med 111: 273–279, 1989.
31. Einzig AI, Wiernik PH, Sasloff J, et al. Phase II study of taxol in patients with advanced ovarian cancer. Proc Am Assoc Cancer Res 31:187, 1990.
31A. Thigeen T, Blessing J, Ball H, et al. Phase II trial of taxol as second-line therapy for ovarian cancer: a Gynecologic Oncology Group Study. Proc Am Soc Clin Oncol 9:156, 1990.
32. Swindell CS, Patel BP, deSolms SJ, et al. A route for the construction of the taxane BC substructure. J Org Chem 52:2346–2355, 1987.
33. Parness J, Kingston GI, Powell RG, et al. Structure-activity study of cytotoxicity and microtubule assembly in vitro by taxol and related taxones. Biochem Biophys Res Commun 105:1082–1089, 1982.
34. Manfredi JJ and Horwitz SB. Taxol: an antimitotic agent with a new mechanism of action. Pharmac Ther 25:83–125, 1984.
35. Masurovsky EB, Peterson ER, Crain SM, et al. Microtubule arrays in taxol-treated mouse dorsal root ganglion-spinal cord cultures. Brain Res 217:392–398, 1981.
36. Masurovsky EB, Peterson ER, Crain SM, et al. Taxol-induced microtubule formations in
37. Masurovsky EB, Peterson ER, Crain SM, et al. Morphologic alterations in dorsal root ganglion neurons and supporting cells of organotypic mouse spinal cord-ganglion cultures exposed to taxol. Neuroscience 10:491–509, 1983.
38. Mole-Bajar J and Bajar AS. Action of taxol on mitosis: Modification of microtubule arrangements and function of the mitotic spindle in hoemanthus endosperm. J Cell Biol 96:527–540, 1983.
39. Letourneau PC and Ressler AH. Inhibition of neurite initiation and growth by taxol. J Cell Biol 98:1355–1362, 1984.
40. Letourneau PC, Shattuck T, Ressler AH. Branching of sensory and sympathetic neurites in vitro is inhibited by treatment with taxol. J neuroscience 6:1912–1917, 1986.
41. Roytta M, Horwitz SB, Raine CS. Taxol induced neuropathy: Short term effects of local injection. J Neurocytology 13:685–701, 1984.
42. Roytta M and Raine CS. Taxol induced neuropathy: Further ultrastructural studies of nerve fiber changes in situ. J Neurocytology 14:157–175, 1985.
43. Roytta M and Raine CS. Taxol induced neuropathy: Chronic effects of local injection. J Neurocytology 15:483–496, 1986.
44. Crain S and Peterson E. Enhanced dependence of fetal mouse neurons on trophic factors after taxol exposure in organotypic cultures. In Cellular and Mollecular Biology of Neuronal Development, IB Block (ed). Plenum Publishing, New York, 1984.
45. Lipton RB, Apfel S, Dutcher JP, et al. Taxol produces a predominantly sensory neuropathy. 39:368–373, 1989.
46. Peterson E and Crain S. Nerve growth factor attenuates neurotoxic effects of taxol on spinal cord-ganglion explants from fetal mice. Science 217:377–379, 1982.
47. Roy SN and Horwitz SB. A phosphoglycoprotein associated with taxol-resistance in J7874.2 cells. Cancer Res 45:3856–3863, 1985.
48. Horwitz SB, Schiff PB, Parness J, et al. Taxol: A Probe for studying the structure and function of microtubules. In: The Cytoskeleton, Clarkson TW (ed). Plenum Publishing, New York, 1986.
49. Horwitz SB, Goei S, Greenberger L, et al. Resistance in the mouse macrophage-like cell line J774-2. In: Mechanisms Of Drug Resistance in Neoplastic Cells, Bristol-Myers Cancer Symposium Vol. 9, PV Woolley III, KD Tew (eds). Academic Press, San Diego, 1988, pp. 223–242.
50. Ling V and Kartner N. Multidrug resistance in cancer. Scient Am 260:44–51, 1989.
51. Gerlach JH, Kartner N, Bell DR, et al. Multidrug resistance. Can Surv 5:25–46, 1986.
52. Pastan I and Gottesman M. Multiple-drug resistance in human cancer. N Engl J Med 316:1388–1393, 1987.

6. ICRF-187 (ADR-529) cardioprotection against anthracycline-induced cardiotoxicity: Clinical and preclinical studies

Michael D. Green, Peggy Alderton, Mordechai M. Sobol, Janet Gross, Franco M. Muggia, and James L. Speyer

Introduction

Anthracyclines are anticancer agents that are effective in a wide range of tumors. Unfortunately, their activity is limited by the development of a chronic dose-dependent cardiomyopathy. The ability of anthracyclines to induce a chronic dose-dependent cardiomyopathy has been well documented. A number of approaches to abrogate this effect have been explored with varying degrees of success. These include the development of analogs of the parent anthracyclines doxorubicin and daunorubicin that retain their antitumor activity but not their cardiotoxic activity; the infusion of anthracyclines over 48–96 hours with considerable diminution of cardiotoxicity and retention of the anticancer effect; and finally, the most successful approach, the development of a specific antagonist of the cardiotoxic effect of anthracycline. The observation that all these approaches have, to varying degrees of success, selectively abrogated the toxic cardiomyopathy caused by anthracyclines without adversely affecting the antitumor response indicates that there must be different mechanisms of anthracycline action, either in different tissues and/or in malignant versus non-malignant cells.

Although the mechanism by which anthracyclines induce cardiotoxicity is only partially understood, there is indirect evidence that doxorubicin stimulates the production of reactive oxygen free radicals in the heart [1–3]. It is believed that free radicals are capable of causing lipid peroxidation of mitochondrial membranes and endoplasmic reticulum [1,3]. Moreover, it would appear that the heart is particularly susceptible to free radical damage, because it has less superoxide dismutase (SOD) and catalase activity than other tissues [4]. This is an observation we have confirmed in our own experiments. Since doxorubicin itself depresses the activity of cardiac glutathione peroxidase (GP) [4], the enzyme that catalyzes the inactivation of lipid peroxides and hydrogen peroxide, there may be an enhanced effect on cardiac damage.

Franco M. Muggia (ed.), NEW DRUGS, CONCEPTS AND RESULTS IN CANCER CHEMOTHERAPY.
 ISBN 0-7923-1253-8

Biochemistry

At present there are basically two biochemical mechanisms that have been proposed to explain anthracycline cardiotoxicity. Until recently the generally accepted theory involved the enzymatic reduction of doxorubicin to a semiquinone radical, which then reduced oxygen to yield oxygen free radicals that initiated lipid peroxidation [1, 2, 5–10]. Recently another hypothesis has evolved in the literature based on the doxorubicin-metal complex, which undergoes redox cycling to produce a powerful oxidant that can cause the degradation of lipids [11–17]. The role of iron in the two hypotheses is a contentious issue, because some investigators query whether in the cell it is present in a high enough concentration to form the reported complex. In the first theory it is required in catalytic amounts to initiate hydroxyl radical production, while in the latter iron forms a complex with drug.

The first hypothesis evolved from work of Handa and Sato [31], who demonstrated that quinone-containing drugs caused an increase in oxygen consumption by liver microsomes. Subsequent work by different groups using microsomal and mitochondrial systems established that electrons are diverted from the proximal end of the electron transport chain at the site of NADPH cytochrome P-450 reductase. The electrons are transferred to the quinone ring of doxorubicin, activating the drug to a semiquinone radical intermediate [1, 5, 18]. Electron spin resonance (ESR) spectroscopy [1, 5] has confirmed that microsomes in the presence of doxorubicin contain the semiquinone radical intermediate. It is now evident that other flavin-containing oxidoreductase enzymes present in the cytoplasm, mitrochondria, sarcoplasmic reticulum, and nuclear membrane are also responsible for activation of anthracyclines to a radical intermediate [19–21]. Under aerobic conditions, such as exists in the myocardial cell, the semiquinone radical donates its unpaired electron to molecular oxygen forming superoxide anions [3, 5, 21, 22]. The generation of superoxide anions by the incubation of microsomes and doxorubicin has been confirmed directly with ESR-spin trapping techniques [23]. The superoxide radical then initiates a cascade of interrelated reactions, which result in the production of hydrogen peroxide [20] and ultimately the hydroxyl radical [24]. In the absence of oxygen, the semiquinone radical may rearrange to form a secondary radical species, which can alkylate DNA and proteins.

Oxygen free radicals are reported to be involved in the stimulation of microsomal [25] and mitochondrial lipid peroxidation [8]. In fact, unsaturated membrane lipids are very susceptible to free radical attack. In particular, the hydroxyl radical, being an extremely reactive species, has been nominated as the most likely candidate to initiate lipid peroxidation. The existence of hydroxyl radicals has been demonstrated in a system composed of doxorubicin and an oxidoreductase enzyme [24]. Doxorubicin enhances lipid peroxidation significantly in heart and liver microsomes [6, 9, 10, 18, 25], and in vivo in the hearts of mice following acute doxorubicin treatment

[2]. Ultrastructural changes observed in the heart after doxorubicin exposure include mitrochondrial degeneration, vacuolization of sacroplasmic reticulum, and disarray of myofilaments, changes indicative of an alternation in membrane structure [26–28]. A number of these authors have speculated that these results all support the contention that lipid peroxidation could be an important mechanism of anthracycline cardiotoxicity.

Free radicals can also directly damage enzymes, other cellular proteins, and nucleic acids. Lipid peroxidation would alter membrane composition, affecting structural integrity, the transport properties of the membrane [26, 29, 30], and the activity of enzymes embedded in the membrane. In addition, the aldehyde degradation products that result from lipid peroxidation are cytotoxic to the cell [32]. These degradation products have been shown to cause functional damage in the cell by reacting with proteins containing sulfydryl groups, causing inactivation of cellular enzymes [33] and inhibiting protein synthesis [34]. Doxorubicin itself appears to directly inhibit mitochondrial and microsomal electron transport enzymes, reducing the energy supply of the heart. Whether cardiotoxicity arises from a single specific effect of doxorubicin metabolism seems unlikely, it is more likely to result from any combination of the effects discussed above.

In the second hypothesis mentioned above, several groups have observed that iron forms a complex with doxorubicin, either as doxorubicin-Fe^{3+} in a 1:3 ratio [11, 35–37] or as a doxorubicin-ADP-Fe^{3+} coordination complex [16, 38], which can cause peroxidation of lipids. Several groups have proposed that iron bound to doxorubicin may be nonenzymatically reduced by internal electron transfer within the complex from Fe^{3+} to Fe^{2+}, which either reduce oxygen to yield oxygen free radicals or themselves act as an oxidant (a perferryl ion) to initiate the breakdown of lipids [2, 12, 37, 38]. A similar mode of action has been postulated for a doxorubicin-copper complex [39]. This theory has been refined by recent structural studies comparing doxorubicin with other anthracycline analogs, enabling a mechanistic model to be proposed [15, 17, 40]. Zweier and coworkers [17] reported, using drug-metal complexes, that doxorubicin was able to reduce bound Fe^{3+}, but daunorubicin was not, unless an exogenous reducing agent was present. A structural comparison of daunorubicin and doxorubicin show that they only differ with respect to one functional side group, a ketone or ketol side chain, respectively. Ketols are more susceptible to oxidation than the corresponding ketones [43]. Thus the mechanism involves initial spontaneous oxidation of the ketol side chain, transferring an electron to the hydroquinone ring to form a semiquinone radical, which then, by electron transfer, reduces chelated Fe^{3+} [17]. The first reduction step may occur either by internal electron transfer or by the interaction between two doxorubicin molecules. This mode of action would explain why doxorubicin is more cardiotoxic than daunorubicin, since the latter drug cannot undergo spontaneous oxidation [15]. Furthermore, changes in the structure or conformation of the amino-sugar component of the anthracycline were shown to result in decreased reduction of bound iron, which correlated with decreased lipid peroxidation. Myers and colleagues [40], using 5-iminodaunomycin, which contains an altered quinone ring structure, demonstrated that this analog was unable to reduce iron. Secondly, due to 5-iminodaunomycin's high affinity for iron, the metal ion was less accessible to reactants, and hence less reactive. These results support the proposal that cardiotoxicity of doxorubicin arises from the ability of the drug's quinone ring to undergo electron transfer in the drug-iron complex. If the quinone ring is altered in any way, the drug becomes less cardiotoxic.

A growing body of evidence questions the involvement of oxygen free radicals in cardiotoxicity. These investigators suggest that the doxorubicin-Fe^{3+} complex itself is a powerful enough oxidant able to initiate lipid peroxidation without the requirement for hydroxyl radicals [15, 36, 38, 41]. In support of this point of view, free radical scavengers were unable to inhibit lipid peroxidation associated with doxorubicin-iron complexes, while iron chelators totally blocked the process [15, 41]. This result suggests that lipid peroxidation is initiated by an oxidant generated by a metal-driven process, rather than by oxygen free radicals. The availability of iron in vivo to form drug-metal complexes has been criticized in the past, suggesting the free iron concentration would not be high enough. However, Demant [42] has shown that doxorubicin can abstract iron from ferritin, the major intracellular storage of iron.

It must be pointed out that all the developmental work for these theories of anthracycline-induced cardiotoxicity have been undertaken in vitro using model systems of microsomes, mitochodria, or reaction mixtures composed of doxorubicin, NADPH, and NADPH cytochrome P-450 reductase. For example, the identification of semiquinone radicals by ESR in microsomal doxorubicin reaction mixtures suggested to the investigators that the drug was enzymatically reduced by microsomal enzymes. However, in retrospect this species may arise from internal electron transfer in a drug-metal complex, rather than reduction by a cellular enzyme. Hence the situation in vivo needs to be confirmed, although this will be a difficult task.

An alternative theory to the free radical hypothesis involves the binding of the negative phospholipid, cardiolipin, and doxorubicin. It has been reported that the drug binds specifically with high affinity to cardiolipin in model membranes [44–46]. Cardiolipin is not simply acting as a receptor for doxorubicin, because the interaction causes a decrease in membrane fluidity, hence altering membrane structure and function [47]. Cardiolipin is normally restricted to mitochondrial membranes, and the heart, being rich in mitochondria, would be a prime target for doxorubciin binding and the associated effects on membrane function [47]. Thus just as oxygen free radicals and associated lipid peroxidation potentially can cause many detrimental effects to membrane function, so could cardiolipin-doxorubicin binding, also leading to cardiac dysfunction.

Why should the heart specifically be susceptible to the damage induced after doxorubicin administration when compared with any other organ in the body? For example, liver microsomes convert doxorubicin to its semiquinone radical at an even greater rate than cardiac microsomes [6, 10] and yet develop none of the clinical damage observed in the heart. The answer probably lies in the biochemical makeup of the heart. The production of oxygen free radicals is a normal part of aerobic cellular metabolism, and so the cell has developed a number of protective antioxidant defenses to remove these species. These antioxidant mechanisms include superoxide dismutase, which dismutates two molecules of superoxide to form hydrogen peroxide and oxygen; catalase, which breaks down hydrogen peroxide to water and oxygen; and the glutathione redox cycle, which removes hydrogen peroxide and other organic peroxides [48, 49]. Reduced glutathione (GSH) in this redox cycle acts as a reductant, removing peroxides, but it can also

Table 1. Enzyme and GSH levels of different organs in mice: Percentage relative to the liver

Organ	SOD Activity	GP Activity	Catalase Activity	GSH Concentration
Heart	42.29 ± 6.47[a]	23.00 ± 7.12	2.90 ± 0.35	25.57 ± 10.55
Kidney	59.00 ± 7.58	129.80 ± 32.23	23.67 ± 6.11	23.50 ± 8.55
Skeletal muscle	17.80 ± 2.86	11.13 ± 3.70	1.37 ± 0.38	9.00 ± 2.55

[a] The percentage value represents the mean ± SD from seven separate experiments, except catalase activity, which was only measured in three experiments. There were three to five mice per treatment group used for each experiment.

Table 2. Effect of doxorubicin on enzyme and GSH levels in several species

Animal	Author(s)	SOD[a]	GP	Catalase	GSH	Model[b]
Mice	51	—	—	—	Dec (35)[c]	Acute
	4	NC	Dec (66)	—	—	Acute
	50	—	—	—	Dec (36)	Acute
	22	Inc (25)	—	Inc (110)	—	Acute
	96	NC	Dec (13)	NC	—	Acute
Rat	64	—	NC	NC	—	Acute
	65[d]	Dec (26)	Inc (14)	—	Dec (46)	Acute
	97	—	Inc (30)	—	Inc (20)	Chronic
Rabbits	52	—	Dec (40)	—	Dec (31)	Chronic
	57	—	NC	NC	Inc (36 chronic 50 acute)	Acute
	98	—	NC	—		Acute/chronic

[a] SOD = superoxide dismutase; GP = glutathione peroxidase; GSH = reduced glutathione.
[b] Animal model, whether doxorubicin was administered by an acute or chronic dose schedule.
[c] NC = no change; dec = decrease; inc = increase. The values in brackets represents the percentage of decrease or increase relative to the control value calculated from published results.
[d] This study used perfused hearts from rats as a model system.

act as a nucleophile, forming thioethers with harmful compounds to detoxify them. We have demonstrated (table 1) that normal levels of these antioxidants in the heart compared with other organs, in particular the liver, are reduced. Based on the observation that the heart has lower levels of superoxide dismutase and reduced glutathione, and very little catalase compared with other organs, it is particularly susceptible to free radical attack.

The effect of doxorubicin on antioxidant levels of the heart has been examined in experimental animal models, summarized in table 2. Based on the results reported in the literature, the effect of doxorubicin on the cardiac antioxidant capacity is variable, depending on the treatment protocol and the species examined. These animal studies suggest that doxorubicin has the potential to alter the cardiac antioxidant capacity, making it even more suspectible to oxygen free radical attack.

Biochemical antagonists of doxorubicin cardiotoxicity

The most promising agents that have been investigated as doxorubicin cardioprotectors in preclinical systems have been two drugs belonging to the bis(dioxopiperazine) family. The two members of this family that are of the most interest and have undergone clinical studies are ICRF 159 and ICRF 187. ICRF 187 is the (+) enantiomer of ICRF 159 and is more water soluble, which allows for better parenteral formulation. These compounds have chelating activity and have a structure similar to ethylene diamine tetraacetic acid (EDTA). They were initially developed as antitumor agents on the hypothesis they may act as intracellular chelating agents and, in fact, did possess cytotoxic activity in vitro. Taylor and Bleehen [53] subsequently showed that ICRF 159 causes cellular arrest and cytotoxicity in the $G_2 + M$ phase of the cell cycle.

Early studies with using dog heart demonstrated that pretreatment with EDTA or ICRF 159 prevented the increase in coronary artery perfusion pressure caused by the anthracyclines [54, 55]. Subsequently it was noted that pretreatment with EDTA or ICRF 159 prevented this increase in coronary artery perfusion pressure [55]. Herman later demonstrated that hamsters given ICRF 159 prior to a high-dose daunorubicin had an increased survival and less acute cardiac toxicity than those treated with daunorubicin alone [56]. Furthermore, in both previous experiments it was noted that plasma and tissue aglycone metabolites were reduced in the ICRF 159-treated animals.

It was initially thought, based on the observation that anthracyclines increase free radical production, that cardioprotection may be offered by reducing the levels of free radicals. With this in mind, several groups utilized free radical scavengers, namely, vitamin E or alpha-tocopherol, N-acetylcysteine, and cysteamine, in combination with the anthracyclines, to see if cardiotoxicity could be reduced. Initial results in several animal models were promising, because acute cardiotoxicity was diminished by these agents [2, 54, 57, 58]. Vitamin E acts by directly scavenging free radicals, while N-acetylcysteine and cysteamine increase the concentration of free sulphydryl groups, enhancing GSH levels and increasing the capacity to detoxify peroxides. However, once studies were extended over longer observation periods, it was reported that chronic cardiotoxicity was not eliminated by these agents [59–63]. Furthermore, under identical experimental conditions comparing vitamin E, N-acetylcysteine, and ICRF-187, only ICRF offered cardioprotection in miniature swine and dogs [59, 61–62]. This result indicates that ICRF-187 is not simply acting as a free radical scavenger, but probably it prevents the formation of oxygen free radicals [59].

There is considerable evidence in animal models to support the role of the bisdioxopiperazines in protecting against doxorubicin cardiotoxicity. Work by Herman et al. with ICRF 187 showed that this isomer of 159 prevented high-dose daunorubicin toxicity in hamsters [60, 66–68]. Wang et al. have demonstrated that the schedule of administration of ICRF 159 is important in prevention of toxicity in mice [69]. They found that the protective effect was maximal when the drug was given between 24 hours prior to and the time of administration of the daunorubicin. Herman et al. [60, 67] have shown that ICRF 187 maximally prevented acute high-dose daunorubicin toxicity in hamsters when the ICRF 187 was administered between 3 hours prior to and 3 hours after the daunorubicin. In a subsequent study, Herman et al. [70] administered ICRF 187 at two dose levels (12.5 mg/kg and 25 mg/kg), 30 minutes prior to daunorubicin, and monitored the cardiac pathological changes. They found highly significant ($p < 0.001$) reductions in anthracycline cardiac pathology in both groups of rabbits pretreated with ICRF 187. Furthermore, they made the interesting observation that the serum iron was reduced in both ICRF 187-treated groups. The ICRF 187 did not add to the systemic toxicity of daunorubicin, as assessed by weight change, myelotoxicity, or serum chemistries. In a randomized study in beagle dogs Herman and Ferrans [71] administered ICRF 187 (12.5 mg/kg) 30 minutes prior to the doxorubicin (1.0 mg/kg), and this schedule was repeated weekly for 15 weeks. This study demonstrated a highly significant difference ($p < 0.001$), with hardly any cardiac pathology occurring in the dogs given ICRF 187. In a subsequent study of miniature swine treated with a 3-weekly schedule of doxorubicin 2.4 mg/kg, with ICRF 187 (12.5 mg/kg) administered 30 minutes prior to the doxorubicin, it was found that the ICRF 187 pretreatment reduced the pathological changes compared to controls ($p = 0.001$) [59, 62].

Clinical studies

Based on the preclinical data described above, which demonstrated cardioprotection by ICRF-187 in a number of species of animals, ranging from rodents to dogs, we decided to test whether these findings could be translated into humans. Despite the fact that ICRF 159 and 187 were inactive as antitumor agents, we believed that preclinical evidence of cardioprotection warranted a clinical trial. We designed a clinical trial to determine whether ICRF-187 could protect humans against anthracycline cardiotoxicity as measured by three distinct and endpoints. Even though Legha and his colleagues [72, 73] had demonstrated that pathological changes characteristic of anthracycline cardiotoxicity accurately predicted for the development of clinical cardiac failure, we decided to introduce the important clinical endpoint of clinical heart failure, as well as a fall in resting left ventricular ejection fraction (LVEF), as measured by sequential MUGA scans. Since the initial observation that ICRF-187-abrogated anthracycline cardiotoxicity was made only on pathology in animals, we believed it was important to correlate the pathologic changes seen in humans with the clinical data. At a cumulative dose of 450 mg/m^2 of doxorubicin, patients were offered a cardiac biopsy, which was read and scored blinded by Dr. Ferrans at the NIH. Since the initial study was reported [74], with 92 patients analyzed, another 50 patients have been entered and are available for analysis.

The study was a prospective randomized trial in women with metastatic breast cancer. Briefly, patients were eligible if they had not received chemotherapy for advanced disease previously, had a resting LVEF more than 0.45, had no active cardiac disease, and had normal bone marrow, liver, and renal function. Following stratification according to prior adjuvant chemotherapy or cardiac risk factors, they were randomized to receive either the combination of doxorubicin 50 mg/m^2, 5-fluorouracil (500 mg/m^2, and cyclophosphamide (500 mg/m^2) (FDC) or the same combination plus ICRF-187. The ICRF-187 was administered as a 1 g/m^2 bolus half an hour prior to the doxorubicin. In both arms all the drugs were administered intravenously and repeated every 3 weeks until either tumor progression occurred or until evidence of cardiac dysfunction was noted. Doxorubicin was not arbitrarily ceased at a predetermined cumulative dose. The cardiac evaluation was performed by the treating oncologists and independently by the study cardiologists and nuclear medicine physicians, neither of whom were informed of the patient's treatment allocation. The MUGA scans were performed prior to the administration of chemotherapy and at cumulative doxorubicin doses of 300 mg/m^2, 450 mg/m^2, and each 100 mg/m^2 thereafter. Antitumor assessments and toxicity grading were scored according to the ECOG criteria [75]. The off-study criteria were unacceptable toxicity (ECOG grade 4), tumor progression, or cardiac toxicity. These latter criteria were the development of clinical heart failure, a fall in the resting LVEF by 0.20 or more, a fall in the resting LVEF to less than 0.45, or an endomyocardial biopsy score rated on the Billingham scale [76] of grade 2 or worse. In an effort to compare the two groups, the fall in LVEF for each patient was calculated from baseline to the subsequent measurement at each of several ranges of cumulative doxorubicin dose. For each dose range, the statistical significance of the difference between the two treatment groups was determined by the rank sum test.

One hundred and forty-two patients were entered into the study. Patient variables, such as age, performance status, poor adjuvant chemotherapy, prior hormone therapy, poor radiation therapy, and cardiac risk factors, were all evenly matched. This analysis includes 112 patients, 89 of whom are off study and can be assessed for cardiac toxicity and antitumor response. Although the median cumulative dose of doxorubicin and the median number of cycles received were higher in the group of patients receiving ICRF-187, this difference did not reach statistical significance. Interestingly, the dose of intensity of both 5-fluorouracil and cyclophosphamide were significantly reduced by a median of about 12%. This was due to our policy of reducing only cyclophosphamide and 5-fluorouracil for hematologic toxicity, so that we would not bias the numbere of cycles of doxorubicin given if the ICRF-187 produced synergistic hematologic toxicity.

There was a convincing effect of ICRF-187 in preventing doxorubicin cardiotoxicity, as demonstrated by the significant difference in fall in resting LVEF when both groups are compared at cumulative doses up to 600 mg/m^2. In fact only one patient who did not have ICRF-187 managed to receive more than 600 mg/m^2, whereas 18 patients who had ICRF-187 received a cumulative dose of doxorubicin of more than 600 mg/m^2. This is reflected in the reasons why patients were removed from the study. Twenty-two of those who received FDC alone had evidence of some form of cardiotoxicity (usually a fall in LVEF), whereas only four receiving ICRF187 had any form of cardiotoxicity ($p < 0.001$). Importantly, six patients on the ICRF-187 arm received more than 1000 mg/m^2 of doxorubicin, whereas none who received FDC alone reached that cumulative dose. There was no evidence that ICRF-187 abrogated the antitumor response of doxorubicin in that the objective response rate (complete remissions and partial remissions) was not significantly different in between arms. It was 45% in the FDC alone arm and 48% in the ICRF-187 arm.

Due to dose reductions built into the trial for hematologic and non-hematologic toxicities, there was no statistical difference between the nadir hematologic counts between the two arms. However, the fact that there was a difference in dose intensity of the 5-fluorouracil and cyclophosphamide suggests that the ICRF-187 contributed to more hematologic (or non-hematologic) toxicity. Although frank congestive cardiac failure was uncommon in this study, mild to moderate failure did occur. Undoubtedly, the relatively high incidence of cardiac failure in this study is due to the stringency of the criteria employed and the aggressiveness with which it was investigated. In the FDC arm there were 11 patients who developed cardiac failure, while in the FDC + ICRF-187 arm there were two ($p < 0.001$). Both episodes in the ICRF-187 were mild, being classified as New York Heart Association grade 1. The endomyocardial biopsy data confirm the findings seen in animals where ICRF-187 provided significant cardioprotection. There were no patients in the ICRF-187 who had a biopsy score of more than 1, whereas there were five patients who had a biopsy score greater than 2 in the FDC arm.

The clinical and the preclinical data presented in this paper confirm the initial hypothesis that ICRF-187 protects against the development of chronic doxorubicin cardiac toxicity. This has now been demonstrated in both humans and numerous animal species. In the preclinical animal studies, the dose of ICRF-187 required for cardiac protection at each treatment course was between 10 and 15 times the dose of doxorubicin [61, 62, 67–71, 77–82]. We chose a dose of 1000 mg/m^2 for ICRF-187, which was 20 times the doxorubicin dose of 50 mg/m^2. This is still considerably lower than the dose of ICRF-187 that caused myelosuppression in the phase I trials [83–87]. When ICRF-187 is added in a dose of 1000 mg/m^2 to this standard doxorubicin-containing regiment, it contributes only a small amount to the major acute toxicity of myelosuppression. Eight percent more 5-fluorouracil and cyclophosphamide were given in the FDC arm. The mean nadir WBC in the first cycle was less in the FDC + ICRF-187 arm, 2.4, compared to 3.0 in the FDC arm. While the dose of ICRF-187 may add a small amount to the myelosuppression of the regimen, this did not significantly result in more fever, infections, or death in that arm of the study.

An obvious concern is whether the addition of ICRF-187 blocks the antitumor activity of the doxorubicin. As indicated previously, there is evidence that antitumor activity of doxorubicin and its cardiac effects may be separable phenomena. In animal studies, cardioprotection by ICRF-187 against chronic doxorubicin-induced pathologic changes was not associated with a reduction in the incidence of other noncardiac toxicity [61, 71]. Furthermore, in vitro studies demonstrated no loss of antitumor activity [88, 89] when the two drugs were combined. The clinical study indicates no differences in the antitumor efficacy of this standard FDC regimen in terms of response rate or time to progression. The objective response rate observed was similar to the rate reported by cooperative groups [90] with the FDC regimen and not unlike most trials in patients with metastatic breast cancers, including failures to adjuvant therapy. Moreover, the time to progression is similar to that reported elsewhere [90]. These results provide confidence that ICRF-187 in this dose does not detract from the activity of the FDC regimen.

The data from the clinical trial is presented with each patient serving as her own control, with the LVEF shown as the change from the patient's own baseline scan. A fall greater than 0.2 certainly represents altered cardiac response, even if it is still in the 'normal' range. A decrease in resting LVEF to less than the normal range is the strongest predictor for clinical toxicity. Nine of 13 patients who had a fall from baseline to less than 0.45 had clinical toxicity (nine FDC and one FDC + ICRF-187). Four of these nine patients receiving FDC only had endomyocardial biopsies. The biopsy scores were 2,

2, 2, and 0.5. Three of these four patients also developed clinical heart failure.

Endomyocardial biopsy is regarded as the most specific and most sensitive measure of doxorubicin cardiac toxicity. Interpretation of the biopsy results is limited by the fact that not all patients who reached a dose of 450 mg/m^2 had biopsies. Fifty-two percent of patients at 450 mg/m^2 in the FDC arm and 48% of patients in the FDC + ICRF arm had biopsies. In the extensive experience with endomyocardial biopsies in patients receiving doxorubicin at Stanford [76] and the MD Anderson [72, 73], scores of 2 or greater are most likely to correlate with major clinical cardiac failure. Of the 13 patients scored as clinically cardiotoxic, only five underwent cardiac biopsies (all on the FDC arm). Biopsy scores of greater than 2 were not observed. Five of 11 evaluable biopsies in the FDC arm had a biopsy score of 2, while none of the 13 patients on the FDC + ICRF-187 arm had a biopsy score of greater than 1. Accepting these limitations, the biopsies showed significant protection by ICRF-187.

One possible mechanism of action of ICRF is suggested by it structure, since it is a nonpolar version of EDTA it can enter myocardial cells and function as an intracellular chelator of divalent cations. As mentioned earlier, iron is intimately associated with anthracycline-induced lipid peroxidation, either acting as a catalyst for production of the hydroxyl radical or by forming a complex with doxorubicin, which then initiates peroxidation. By chelating iron ICRF could prevent these two possible modes of action of cardiotoxicity. To support the theory that ICRF chelates iron, it has been reported that ICRF-159 passively diffuses through cells membranes, where it is hydrolyzed to a product (ICRF-198) that strongly binds iron, abstracting it from a doxorubicin-iron complex [91]. In addition ICRF-187 increases the renal clearance of iron, copper, and other transition metal ions [86]. Myers and coworkers [11] reported that EDTA removed iron from the doxorubicin-iron complex and completely blocked lipid peroxidation of the membranes by the drug-metal complex. Furthermore, ICRF-187 has been demonstrated to prevent another disease with a proposed iron-catalyzed free radical mechanism of tissue toxicity, alloxon-induced diabetes in mice [92, 93]. It is postulated that alloxan increases the production of free radicals, in particular, the hydroxyl radical formed by an iron-catalyzed mechanism, which destroys the pancreatic beta-cell, resulting in hyperglycemia [94]. It is thought ICRF-187 attenuates hyperglycemia by preventing the formation of hydroxyl radicals through iron chelation [93].

Thus, based on the etiology of anthracycline cardiotoxicity, ICRF could be offering cardioprotection by preventing the formation of either the semiquinone intermediate, the oxygen free radicals, or the doxorubicin-iron complex. In this role ICRF would be acting as an iron chelator. Alternatively, ICRF may alter the balance in the cardiac antioxidant defense mechanism, thereby abrogating any depression induced by doxorubicin and enabling the heart to counteract an increase in free radicals.

It is important to point out that ICRF does not affect the antitumor activity of anthracycline drugs [2, 81, 82]. Also, other anthracycline-induced toxicities, such as alopecia and bone marrow suppression, were unaffected by combination treatment with ICRF [56, 62, 95]. In fact, Woodman and coworkers [81] reported that the effectiveness of doxorubicin or daunorubicin against L120 leukaemia in mice was enhanced in combination with ICRF-159, associated with a reduction in the cardiotoxicity for daunorubicin but not doxorubicin. Employing the murine sarcoma S180 cell line, we demonstrated previously that the addition of ICRF-187 to doxorubicin synergistically inhibits the ability of tumor cells to proliferate in liquid medium [89]. In an effort to evaluate the effects of the combination of doxorubicin and ICRF-187 on S180 cell-cycle traverse, we employed flow microfluorometry to analyze cell DNA content following 24-hour exposure to drug. To determine whether the antiproliferative effects of the drug combination represent primary lethal events or sublethal cytostatic effects, the results of flow cytometry were compared with colony-forming efficiency. Twenty-four hour incubation with either agent produced dose-dependent partial G_2M arrest. At high doses, ICRF-187 produced partial G_2M arrest, inhibition of cell division, and continued DNA synthesis at a higher ploidy, resulting in a second G_2M arrest of an 8n population. The addition of ICRF-187 to doxorubicin resulted in enhancement of cell-cycle blockade at G_2M. We subsequently demonstrated that the combination also produced enhanced lethality, as measured by reduced colony-forming efficiency of drug-treated S180 cells [88]. Measurement of doxorubicin accumulated in, and effux from, ICRF-187-pretreated cells failed to reveal an effect of pretreatment with the bis-dioxopiperazine on anthracycline disposition by S180 cells, suggesting that the enhanced cytotoxic and cytostatic effects do not result from increased intracellular concentrations of doxorubicin [88]. We concluded that the positive interaction between the two drugs represented site-specific enhancement of the anthracycline effect by ICRF-187 at an intracellular target site.

In conclusion, ICRF-187 has proven to be a very effective cardioprotector in clinical trials, overcoming the problem of doxorubicin cardiotoxicity without affecting antitumor activity. The mechanism of cardioprotection is not understood, however, it is possible that it chelates iron, preventing the induction of oxygen free radicals by doxorubicin or a doxorubicin-iron complex. If this theory proves to be correct, ICRF-187 has the potential to act as a protective agent against any toxicity that is caused by iron-catalyzed oxygen free-radical generation.

Acknowledgments

This study was supported by the Anti-Cancer Council of Victoria, PHS grants CA 36524, CA 16087, and CRC-RR-99.

References

1. Bachur NR, Gordon SL, and Gee MV. A general mechanism for microsomal activation of quinone anticancer agents to free radicals. Cancer Res 38:1745–1750, 1978.
2. Myers CE, McGuire WP, Liss RH, Ifrim I, et al. Adriamycin: the role of lipid peroxidation in cardiac toxicity and tumor response. Science 197:165–167, 1977.
3. Thayer WS. Adriamycin stimulated superoxide formation in submitochondrial particles. Chem-Biol Inter 19:265–278, 1977.
4. Doroshow JH, Locker GY, and Myers CE. Enzymatic defenses of the mouse heart against reactive oxygen metabolites. J Clin Invest 65:128–135, 1980.
5. Bachur NR, Gordon SL, and Gee MV. Anthracycline antibiotic augmentation of microsomal electron transport and free radical formation. Mol Pharmacol 13:901–910, 1977.
6. Mimnaugh EG, Gram TE, and Trush MA. Stimulation of mouse heart and liver microsomal lipid peroxidation by anthracycline anticancer drugs: characterization and effects of reactive oxygen scavengers. J Pharmacol Exp Ther 226:806–816, 1983.
7. Mimnaugh EG, Kennedy KA, Trush MA, and Sinha BK. Adriamycin-enhanced membrane lipid peroxidation in isolated rat nuclei. Cancer Res 45:3296–3304, 1985.
8. Mimnaugh EG, Trush MA, Bhatnagar M, and Gram TE. Enhancement of reactive oxygen-dependent mitochondrial membrane lipid peroxidation by the anticancer drug adriamycin. Biochem Pharmacol 34:847–856, 1985.
9. Mimnaugh EG, Trush MA, Ginsburg E, and Gram TE. Differential effects of anthracycline drugs on rat heart and liver microsomal reduced nicotinamide adenine dinucleotide phosphate-dependent lipid peroxidation. Cancer Res 42:3574–3582, 1982.
10. Mimnaugh EG, Trush MA, and Gram TE. Enhancement of rat heart microsomal lipid peroxidation following doxorubicin treatment in vivo. Cancer Treat Rep 67:731–733, 1983.
11. Myers CE, Gianna L, Simone CB, Klecker R, and Greene R. Oxidative destruction of erythrocyte ghost membranes catalyzed by the doxorubicin-iron complex. Biochemistry 21:1707–1713, 1982.
12. Gianni L, Zweier JL, Levy A, and Myers CE. Characterization of the cycle of iron-mediated electron transfer from Adriamycin to molecular oxygen. J Biol Chem 260:6820–6826, 1985.
13. Muindi J, Sinha BK, Gianni L, and Myers C. Thiol-dependent DNA damage produced by anthracycline-iron complexes. The structure-activity relationships and molecular mechanisms. Mol Pharmacol 27:356–365, 1985.
14. Muindi JR, Sinha BK, Gianni L, and Myers CE. Hydroxyl radical production and DNA damage induced by anthracycline-iron complex. FEBS Lett 172:226–230, 1984.
15. Gianna L, Vigano L, Lanzi C, et al. Role of daunosamine and hydroxyacetyl side chain in reaction with iron and lipid peroxidation by anthracyclines. J Natl Cancer Inst 80:1104–1111, 1988.
16. Sugioka K, Nakano H, Nakano M, et al. Generation of hydroxyl radicals during the enzymatic reductions of the Fe^{3+}-ADP-phosphate-Adriamycin and Fe^{3+}-ADP-EDTA systems. Biochem Biophys Acta 753:411–421, 1983.
17. Zweier JL, Gianni L, Muindi J, and Myers CE. Differences in O_2 reduction by the iron complexes of adriamycin and daunomycin: the importance of the sidechain hydroxyl group. Biochim Biophys Acta 884:326–336, 1986.
18. Goodman J and Hochstein P. Generation of free radicals and lipid peroxidation by redox cycling of Adriamycin and daunomycin. Biochem Biophys Res Commun 77:797–803, 1977.
19. Doroshow JH and Davies KJ. Redox cycling of anthracyclines by cardiac mitochondria. II Formation of superoxide anion, hydrogen peroxide, and hydroxyl radical. J Biol Chem 261:3068–3074, 1986.
20. Davies KJ and Doroshow JH. Redox cycling of anthracyclines by cardiac mitochondria. I Anthracycline radical formation by NADH dehydrogenase. J Biol Chem 261:3060–3067, 1986.

21. Doroshow JH. Effect of anthracycline antibiotics on oxygen radical formation in rat heart. Cancer Res 43:460–472, 1983.
22. Adachi T, Nagae T, Ito Y, Hirano K, and Sugiura M. Relation between cardiotoxic effect of Adriamycin and superoxide anion radical. J Pharm Dyn 6:114–123, 1983.
23. Myers CE. Role of iron in anthracycline action. In: Organ Directed Toxicities of Anticancer Drugs, Hacker MP, Lazo JS, and Tritton TR (eds). Martinus Nijhoff Publishing, Boston, 1988, pp. 17–30.
24. Komiyama T, Kikuchi T, and Sugiura Y. Generation of hydroxyl radical by anticancer quinone drugs, carbazilquinone, mitomycin C, aclacinomycin A and adriamycin, in the presence of NADPH-cytochrome P-450 reductase. Biochem Pharmacol 31:3651–3656, 1982.
25. Mimnaugh EG, Trush MA, and Gram TE. Stimulation by Adriamycin of rat heart and liver microsomal NADH-dependent lipid peroxidation. Biochem Pharmacol 30:2797–2804, 1981.
26. Olson HM and Capen CC. Subacute cardiotoxicity of Adriamycin in the rat. Lab Invest 37:386–394, 1977.
27. Young DM. Pathologic effects of Adriamycin in experimental systems. Can Chemother Rep 6(Part 3):159–175, 1975.
28. Jaenke RS. An anthracycline antibiotic-induced cardiomyopathy in rabbits. Lab Invest 30:292–304, 1974.
29. Maridonneau I, Braquet P, and Garay RP. Na^+ and K^+ transport damage induced by oxygen free radicals in human red cell membranes. J Biol Chem 258:3107–3113, 1983.
30. Sies H, Graf P, and Estrela JM. Hepatic calcium efflux during cytochrome P-450-dependent drug oxidations at the endoplasmic reticulum in intact liver. Proc Natl Acad Sci USA 78:3358–3362, 1981.
31. Handa K, and Sato S. Stimulation of microsomal NADPH oxidation by quinone-group containing anticancer chemicals. Gann 67:523–528, 1976.
32. Benedetti A, Comporti M, Fulceri R, and Esterbauer H. Cytotoxic aldehydes originating from the peroxidation of liver microsomal lipids. Identification of 4,5-dihydroxydecenal. Biochim Biophys Acta 792:172–181, 1984.
33. Benedetti A, Casini AF, Ferrali M, and Comporti M. Effects of diffusible products of peroxidation of rat liver microsomal lipids. Biochem J 180:303–312, 1979.
34. Benedetti A, Barbieri L, Ferrali M, Casini AF, Fulceri R, and Comporti M. Inhibition of protein synthesis by carbonyl compounds (4-hydroxyalkenals) originating from the peroxidation of liver microsomal lipids. Chem Biol Interact 35:331–340, 1981.
35. May PM, Williams GK, and Williams DR. Solution chemistry studies of adriamycin—iron complexes present in vivo. Eur J Cancer 16:1275–1276, 1980.
36. Gutteridge JMC. Adriamycin-iron catalyzed phospholipid peroxide: A reaction not involving reduced Adriamycin or hydroxyl radicals. Biochem Pharmacol 32:1949–1952, 1983.
37. Gutteridge JMC. Lipid peroxidation and possible hydroxyl radical formation stimulated by the self-reduction of a doxorubicin-iron(III) complex. Biochem Pharmacol 33:1725–1728, 1984.
38. Sugioka K and Nakano M. Mechanisms of phospholipid peroxidation induced by ferric ion-ADP Adriamycin coordination complex. Biochem Biophys Acta 713:333–343, 1982.
39. Wallace KB and Johnson JA. Oxygen-dependent effect of microsomes on the binding of doxorubicin to rat hepatic nuclear DNA. Mol Pharmacol 31:307–311, 1987.
40. Myers CE, Muindi JR, Zweier J, and Sinha BK. 5-Iminodaunomycin. An anthracycline with unique properties. J Biol Chem 262:11571–11577, 1987.
41. Minotti G and Aust SD. The requirement for iron(III) in the initiation of lipid peroxidation by iron(II) and hydrogen peroxide. J Biol Chem 262:1098–1104, 1987.
42. Demant EJ. Transfer of ferritin-bound iron to adriamycin. FEBS Lett 176:97–100, 1984.
43. Finkelstein E, Rosen GM, and Rauckman EJ. Production of hydroxyl radical by decomposition of superoxide spin-trapped adducts. Mol Pharmacol 21:262–265, 1982.
44. Duarte-Karim M, Ruysschaert JM, and Hildebrand J. Affinity of Adriamycin to phos-

pholipids. A possible explantion for cardiac mitochondrial lesions. Biochem Biophys Res Comm 71:658–663, 1976.
45. Goormagtigh E, Chatelain P, Caspers J, and Russchaert JM. Evidence of a specific complex between Adriamycin and negatively-charged phospholipids. Biochem Biophys Acta 597:1–14, 1980.
46. Goormaghtigh E, Chatelain P, Caspers J, and Ruysschaert JM. Evidence of a complex between adriamycin derivatives and cardiolipin: possible role in cardiotoxicity. Biochem Pharmacol 29:3003–3010, 1980.
47. Tritton TR, Murphree SA, and Sartorelli AC. Adriamycin: a proposal on the specificity of drug action. Biochem Biophys Res Commun 84:802–808, 1978.
48. Arrick BA and Nathan CF. Glutathione metabolism as a determinant of therapeutic efficacy: a review. Cancer Res 44:4224–4232, 1984.
49. Arrick BA, Nathan CF, and Cohn ZA. Inhibition of glutathione synthesis augments lysis of murine tumor cells by sulfhydryl-reactive antineoplastics. J Clin Invest 71:258–267, 1983.
50. Olson RD, Macdonald JS, Van Boxtel CJ, Harbison RD, Slonium AE, Freeman RW, and Boerth RC. Regulatory role of glutathione and soluble sulfhydryl groups in the toxicity of Adriamycin. J Pharmacol Exp Ther 215:450–454, 1980.
51. Doroshow JH, Locker GY, Baldinger J, and Myers CE. The effect of doxorubicin on hepatic and cardiac glutathione. Res Comm Path Pharmacol 26:285–295, 1979.
52. Revis NW and Marusic N. Glutathione peroxidase activity and selenium concentration in the hearts of doxorubicin-treated rabbits. J Mol Cell Cardiol 10:945–951, 1978.
53. Taylor IW, and Bleehen NM. Razoxane-induced polyploidy. Br J Cancer 38:143–147, 1978.
54. Doroshow JH, Locker GY, Ifrim I, and Myers CE. Prevention of doxorubicin cardiac toxicity in the mouse by N-acetylcysteine. J Clin Invest 68:1053–1064, 1981.
55. Herman EH, Mhatre RM, Lee IP, and Waravdekar VS. Prevention of the cardiotoxic effects of adriamycin and daunorubicin in the isolated dog heart. Proc Soc Exp Biol Med 140:234–249, 1972.
56. Herman EH, Mhatre RM, and Chadwick DP. Modification of some of the toxic effects of daunomycin (NSC-82151) by pretreatment with the antineoplastic agent ICRF-159 (NSC-129943). Toxicol Appl Pharmacol 27:517–526, 1974.
57. Wang Y-M, Madanat FF, Kimball JC, Gleiser CA, Ali MD, Kaufman MW, and Van Eys J. Effect of vitamin E against Adriamycin-induced toxicity in rabbits. Cancer Res 40: 1022–1027, 1980.
58. Sonneveld P. Effect of alpha-tocopherol on the cardiotoxicity of adriamycin in the rat. Cancer Treat Rep 62:1033–1036, 1978.
59. Herman EH and Ferrans VJ. Amelioration of chronic anthracycline cardiotoxicity by ICRF-187 and other compounds. Cancer Treat Rev 14:225–229, 1987.
60. Herman EH, el-Hage AN, Creighton AM, Witiak DT, and Ferrans VJ. Comparison of the protective effect of ICRF-187 and structurally related analogues against acute daunorubicin toxicity in Syrian golden hamsters. Res Commun Chem Pathol Pharmacol 48:39–55, 1985.
61. Herman EH, Ferrans VJ, Myers CE, and Van Vleet JF. Comparison of the effectiveness of (+/−)-1,2-bis(3,5-dioxopiperazinyl-1-yl)propane (ICRF-187) and N-acetylcysteine in preventing chronic doxorubicin cardiotoxicity in beagles. Cancer Res 45:276–281, 1985.
62. Herman EH and Ferrans VJ. Influence of vitamin E and ICRF-187 on chronic doxorubicin cardiotoxicity in miniature swine. Lab Invest 49:69–77, 1983.
63. Breed JG, Zimmerman AN, Dormans JA, and Pinedo HM. Failure of the antioxidant vitamin E to protect against adriamycin-induced cardiotoxicity in the rabbit. Cancer Res 40:2033–2038, 1980.
64. Porta EA, Joun NS, Matsumura L, Nakasone B, and Sablan H. Acute adriamycin cardiotoxicity in rats. Res Comm Chem Path Pharmac 41:125–137, 1983.
65. Julicher RHM, Sterrenberg L, Bast A, Rikensen ROWM, Koomen JM, and Noorheok J. The role of lipid peroxidation in acute doxorubicin-induced cardiotoxicity as studied in rat

isolated heart. J Pharm Pharmacol 38:277–282, 1986.
66. el-Hage AN, Herman EH, and Ferrans VJ. Examination of the protective effect of ICRF-187 and dimethyl sulfoxide against acetaminophen-induced hepatotoxicity in Syrian golden hamsters. Toxicology 28:295–303, 1983.
67. Herman EH, el-Hage AN, Ferrans VJ, and Witiak DT. Reduction by ICRF-187 of acute daunorubicin toxicity in Syrian golden hamsters. Res Commun Chem Pathol Pharmacol 40:217–231, 1983.
68. Herman E, Ardalan B, Bier C, Waravdekar V, and Krop S. Reduction of daunorubicin lethality and myocardial cellular alterations by pretreatment with ICRF-187 in Syrian golden hamsters. Cancer Treat Rep 63:89–92, 1979.
69. Wang G, Finch MD, Trevan D, and Hellmann K. Reduction of daunomycin toxicity by razoxane. Br J Cancer 43:871–877, 1981.
70. Herman EH, Ferrans VJ, Jordan W, and Ardalan B. Reduction of chronic daunorubicin cardiotoxicity by ICRF-187 in rabbits. Res Commun Chem Pathol Pharmacol 31:85–97, 1981.
71. Herman EH and Ferrans VJ. Reduction of chronic doxorubicin cardiotoxicity in dogs by pretreatment with (+/−)-1,2-bis(3,5-dioxopiperazinyl-1-yl)propane (ICRF-187). Cancer Res 41:3436–3440, 1981.
72. Legha SS, Benjamin RS, Mackay B, Yap HY, Wallace S, Ewer M, Blumenschein GR, and Freireich EJ. Adriamycin therapy by continuous intravenous infusion in patients with metastatic breast cancer. Cancer 49:1762–1766, 1982.
73. Legha SS, Benjamin RS, Mackay B, Ewer M, Wallace S, Valdivieso M, Rasmussen SL, Blumenschein GR, and Freireich EJ. Reduction of doxorubicin cardiotoxicity by prolonged continuous intravenous infusion. Ann Intern Med 96:133–139, 1982.
74. Speyer JL, Green MD, Kramer E, Rey M, Sanger J, Ward C, Dubin N, Ferrans V, Stecy P, Jacquotte-Zeleniuch A, Wernz J, Feit F, Slater W, Blum R, and Muggia F. Protective effect of the bispiperazinedione ICRF-187 against doxorubicin-induced cardiac toxicity in women with advanced breast cancer. N Engl J Med 319:745–752, 1988.
75. Oken MM, Creech RH, Tormey DC, Horton J, Davis TE, McFadden ET, and Carbone PP. Toxicity and response criteria of the Eastern Cooperative Oncology Group. Am J Clin Oncol 5:649–655, 1982.
76. Bristow MR, Mason JW, Billingham ME, et al. Doxorubicin cardiomyopathy: Evaluation by phonocardiography, endomyocardial biopsy, and cardiac catheterization. Ann Intern Med 88:168–175, 1978.
77. Perkins WE, Schroeder RL, Carrano RA, and Imondi AR. Effect of ICRF-187 on doxorubicin-induced myocardial effects in the mouse and guinea pig. Br J Cancer 46:662–667, 1982.
78. Herman EH, el-Hage A, and Ferrans VJ. Protective effect of ICRF-187 on doxorubicin-induced cardiac and renal toxicity in spontaneously hypertensive (SHR) and normotensive (WKY) rats. Toxicol Appl Pharmacol 92:42–53, 1988.
79. Wheeler RH, Clauw DJ, Natale RB, and Ruddon RW. The cytokinetic and cytotoxic effects of ICRF-159 and ICRF-187 in vitro and ICRF-187 in human bone marrow in vivo. Invest New Drugs 1:283–295, 1983.
80. Creighton AM, Hellmann K, and Whitecross S. Antitumour activity in a series of bis-diketopiperazines. Nature 222:384–385, 1969.
81. Woodman RJ, Cysyk RL, Kline I, Gang M, and Vendetti JM. Enhancement of the effectiveness of daunorubicin (NSC-82151) or adriamycin (NSC-123127) against early mouse L1210 leukemia with ICRF-159 (NSC-129943). Cancer Chemother Rep 59:689–695, 1975.
82. Giuliani F, Casazza AM, Di Marco A, and Savi G. Studies in mice treated with ICRF-159 combined with daunorubicin or doxorubicin. Cancer Treat Rep 65:267–276, 1981.
83. Koeller JM, Earhart RH, and Davis HL. Phase I trial of ICRF-187 by 48-hour continuous infusion. Cancer Treat Rep 65:459–463, 1981.

84. Earhart RH, Tutsch KD, Koeller JM, Rodriguez R, Robins HI, Vogel CL, Davis HL, and Tormey DC. Pharmacokinetics of (+)-1,2-di(3,5-dioxopiperazin-1-yl)propane intravenous infusions in adult cancer patients. Cancer Res 42:5255–5261, 1982.
85. Liesmann J, Belt R, Haas C, and Hoogstraten B. Phase I evaluation of ICRF-187 (NSC-169780) in patients with advanced malignancy. Cancer 47:1959–1962, 1981.
86. Von Hoff DD, Howser D, Lewis BJ, Holcenberg J, Weiss RB, and Young RC. Phase I study of ICRF-187 using a daily for 3 days schedule. Cancer Treat Rep 65:249–252, 1981.
87. Holcenberg JS, Tutsch KD, Earhart RH, Ungerleider RS, Kamen BA, Pratt CB, Gribble TJ, and Glaubiger DL. Phase I study of ICRF-187 in pediatric cancer patients and comparison of its pharmacokinetics in children and adults. Cancer Treat Rep 70:703–709, 1986.
88. Wadler S, Green MD, Basch R, and Muggia FM. Lethal and sublethal effects of the combination of doxorubicin and the bisdioxopiperazine, (+)-1,2,-bis(3-5-dioxopiperazinyl-1-yl)propane (ICRF 187), on murine sarcoma S180 in vitro. Biochem Pharmacol 36:1495–1501, 1987.
89. Wadler S, Green MD, and Muggia FM. Synergistic activity of doxorubicin and the bisdioxopiperazine (+)-1,2-bis(3,5-dioxopiperazinyl-1-yl)propane (ICRF 187) against the murine sarcoma S180 cell line. Cancer Res 46:1176–1181, 1986.
90. Henderson IC and Canellos GP. Cancer of the breast: the past decade (first of two parts). N Engl J Med 302:17–30, 1980.
91. Hasinoff BB. The interaction of the cardioprotection agent ICRF-187((+)-1-2-bis(3,5-dioxopiperazinyl-1-yl)propane); its hydrolysis product(ICRF-198); and other chelating agents with the Fe(III) and Cu(II) complexes of adriamycin. Agents Actions 26:378–385, 1989.
92. el-Hage AN, Herman EH, and Ferrans VJ. Reduction in the diabetogenic effect of alloxan in mice by treatment with the antineoplastic agent ICRF-187. Res Commun Chem Pathol Pharmacol 33:509–523, 1981.
93. el-Hage A, Herman EH, Yang GC, Crouch RK, and Ferrans VJ. Mechanism of the protective activity of ICRF-187 against alloxan-induced diabetes in mice. Res Commun Chem Pathol Pharmacol 52:341–360, 1986.
94. Fischer LJ and Hamburger SA. Inhibition of alloxan action in isolated pancreatic islets by superoxide dismutase, catalase, and a metal chelator. Diabetes 29:213–216, 1980.
95. Herman EH, Ferrans VJ, Bhat HB, and Witiak DT. Reduction of chronic doxorubicin cardiotoxicity in beagle dogs by bis-morpholinomethyl derivative of razoxane (ICRF-159). Cancer Chemother Pharmacol 19:277–281, 1987.
96. Kanter MM, Hamlin RL, Unverferth DV, Davis HW, and Merolda AJ. Effect of exercise training on antioxidant enzymes and cardiotoxicity of doxorubicin. J Appl Physiol 59:1298–1303, 1985.
97. Thayer WS. Investigation of the role of serum lipoprotein-associated peroxides in Adriamycin cardiotoxicity. Release of reduced glutathione from rat hearts perfused with lipase-hydrolyzed very low density lipoprotein fractions obtained from Adriamycin-treated and control rats. Biochem Pharmac 38:1923–1929, 1989.
98. Jackson JA, Reeves JP, Muntz KH, Kruk D, Prough RA, Willerson JT, and Buja LM. Evaluation of free radical effects and catecholamine alterations in adriamycin cardiotoxicity. Am J Path 117:140–153, 1984.

7. Uroprotection in patients receiving cyclophosphamide and ifosfamide

Nikhil C. Munshi, Patrick J. Loehrer, and Stephen D. Williams

Introduction

In recent times the development of chemotherapeutic agents with totally new structures and novel modes of action has not been very successful. In the absence of success in this very important direction, pharmacological research has concentrated on variations in the use of the presently known agents. Structural analogs of these chemotherapeutic agents are synthesized to create agents with lesser toxicity or higher potency or both. Pharmacologically designed drug combinations with differing sites of action and protocols with increased dose intensity are showing some promise. One recent innovation has been designing agents that are pharmacologically noncytotoxic but control or prevent toxic side effects of an administered cytotoxic agent. These protective agents allow administration of presently available agents at much higher doses.

Cyclophosphamide and its analogue ifosfamide are both widely used oxazaphosphorine cytostatics. They are effective against many tumors and are relatively well tolerated; a major toxicity is urothelial. Hemorrhagic cystitis is the dose-limiting factor for these agents. This adverse effect described by Philips et al. [1] depends to an extent on drug dosage, concomitant medication, and preexisting urologic disease. Increased toxicity has been reported with prolonged administration in usual doses or a higher single dose [2]; prior or simultaneous radiation to the bladder area [3]; and simultaneous treatment with cisplatin, melphalan, or methotrexate [4,5]. With high-dose regimens, more than 40% of patients showed urotoxicity and a 4% mortality rate from massive bladder hemorrhage, even with vigorous hydration [1,6,7]. To prevent this dose-limiting toxicity, regional detoxification with various thiol compounds has been attempted. The pharmacological aspects and the role of thiols in uroprotection are described below.

Franco M. Muggia (ed.), NEW DRUGS, CONCEPTS AND RESULTS IN CANCER CHEMOTHERAPY.

ISBN 0-7923-1253-8

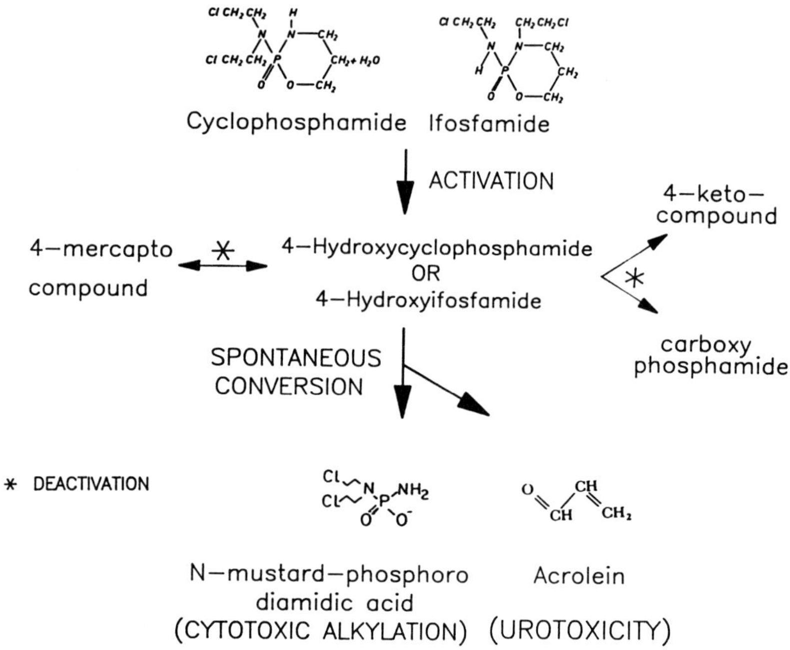

Figure 1. Metabolism of cyclophosphamide or ifosfamide.

Pharmacology of oxazaphosphorines

Oxazaphosphorine cytostatics, in general, and cyclophosphamide and ifosfamide, in particular, are inactive in their parent form. They undergo biotransformation before they become cytocidal. The metabolism is divided into three stages [8, 9], as shown in figure 1. The initial activation takes place by hydroxylation, forming 4-hydroxy cyclophosphamide (4-OH-CP) or ifosfamide (4-OH-IFO). This more reactive metabolite undergoes spontaneous conversion, forming the main alkylating product, nitrogen mustard phosphoro diamidic acid and acrolein. The activation and spontaneous reactions are rate limiting, and hence deactivated intermediates are produced by reversible or irreversible reactions. Less than 10% of drug may also undergo enzymatic side-chain oxidation in liver and kidney, with formation of chloroacetaldehyde [10]. The side-chain oxidation is quantitatively more important in ifosfamide than cyclophosphamide [11].

The reactive aldehyde, acrolein, is a noncytotoxic metabolic product, which causes urothelial toxicity. Acrolein is produced in circulating blood, cells, and urine. Blood and most cells in the body contain thiol compounds, such as glutathione or cysteine, which deactivate toxic reactive chemicals. Acrolein produced in the cell or circulation is inactivated by these thiols, hence sparing the majority of organs in the body of its toxic effects. Acrolein excreted in urine or produced in urine after excretion of the 4-hydroxy metabolite of cyclophosphamide or ifosfamide has a different metabolic fate. The level of the protective thiols are very low in the ureter and bladder. The longer exposure of these organs to acrolein, which is five to ten times more reactive than the 4-hydroxy metabolites, leads to local reaction. They cause concentration-dependent renal pelvic, ureter, and bladder irritation and inflammation. The role of choloracetaldehyde in the pathogenesis of this side effect is postulated but is not clearly proven.

Biological rationale for uroprotection

Administration of cyclophosphamide or ifosfamide leads to a dose-dependent incidence of hemorrhagic cystitis. The incidence of hemorrhagic cystitis with cyclophosphamide ranges from 0 to 50% [12, 13], while the incidence with ifosfamide ranges from 20 to 30% for a lower dose range of 600–1200 mg/m^2 [14, 15] and up to 50–100% with higher doses [16–18] and standard prophylactic measures, including hydration, diuresis, bladder irrigation, and alkalinization of urine. Instillation of locally active compounds into bladder was also tried to prevent this urotoxicity, with minor advantage. The efficacy and practicability of these standard and essentially local measures remain unsatisfactory. Thus the use of systemically administered chemical agents with the ability to inactivate the reactive metabolites was investigated.
reactive metabolites was investigated.

Thiols with their sulfhydryl-SH group bind with reactive species and stabilize the reactive compound. If this occurs in circulation or intracellularly, the chemotherapeutic agent might be rendered less effective. The ideal systemic uroprotector should bind the oxazaphosphorine or its metabolites only in the urine, be nontoxic, be effective when administered systemically, and should not affect the chemotherapeutic potential of the compound. Ideally the agent should be inactive in circulation and be activated only in the urinary tract.

Different thiols were tried and N-acetylcystein (NAC) was one of the first agents used in this manner. Its initial use was as a locally instilled detoxifying agent. This method was only partially successful, and it did not protect the renal pelvis and ureter from urothelial toxicity. NAC has a wide systemic distribution when given orally and will bind oxazaphosphorine metabolites in the tissues and circulation. Conceivably this might lessen the activity of the oxazaphosphorines. Only 15% of the oral dose of NAC is excreted in urine, and thus large doses are required. However, in the absence of better agents, NAC was used clinically to prevent urothelial toxicity with high-dose oxazaphosphorine therapy.

In 1979 Scheef [19] showed preliminary data suggesting the effectiveness of 2-mercaptoethanesulfonate (mesna) as a uroprotective agent. Further studies have shown this agent to be superior to all other agents for uroprotection [20].

Pharmacology of mesna

After entering the circulation, mesna undergoes autooxidation into its disulfide form, dimesna, which is inactive, stable, and unable to enter cells. More than 90% of mesna remains in the dimesna form in circulation [21]. It is rapidly transported to the kidney without getting concentrated in any organ in the body. In the renal tubule it is reduced to mesna, and free thiol becomes available in urine to react with oxazaphosphorine metabolites, and the reaction involves oxidation of glutathione. In the circulation mesna also forms disulfide bond with cysteine and increases its excretion in urine. Cysteine can also act as a free thiol in urine to inactivate acrolein. This mechanism prevents systemic detoxification of oxazaphosphorines and allows local deactivation without interfering with their systemic activity. Scheulen et al. treated 60 testicular cancer patients with ifosfamide, of whom 27 received standard prophylaxis while 33 received mesna. There was no difference in their response rates [22].

Renal conversion of mesna makes its protective action available from the renal pelvis to ureter and bladder. Mesna in urine binds directly to the double bond of acrolein, forming a stable thiol adduct. It also decreases the spontaneous conversion of 4-hydroxy metabolites of oxazaphosphorines by forming stable products with them.

Intravenously administered mesna is converted into its disulfide form within minutes. Its half-life in the blood is 1.5 hours, and it is detected in urine in free thiol form for more than 4 hours. Orally administered mesna is absorbed primarily in the large intestine and, due to a delay in absorption, has a longer half-life [23, 24]. There are no drug interaction with mesna, except that it is physically incompatible with cisplatin and hence should not be mixed with this agent. Mesna does not have significant toxicity, even at very high doses.

Clinical uses and dosages

As seen in table 1, patients receiving ifosfamide and either standard or mesna prophylaxis showed a significant reduction in the incidence of hematuria with mesna.

The relative effectiveness of NAC and mesna as uroprotective agents was compared in a group of testicular cancer patients receiving cisplatin and ifosfamide as salvage chemotherapy at Indiana University. Due to the unavailability of mesna, the initial 80 patients received NAC as a uroprotector at a dose of 2.0 g orally at a q6h dose, while the subsequent 149 patients received mesna as an initial bolus of 10% of the ifosfamide dose; followed by a 24-hour infusion at a dose equal to the ifosfamide dose, which was 0.9–1.2 g/m^2 daily for 5 days. Twenty-four of the 80 patients (30%) receiving NAC developed hematuria, while only 5 out of 149 patients (3.4%) receiving

Table 1. Comparison of standard versus mesna prophylaxis in patients receiving ifosfamide

	Frequency of Hematuria		
No.	Mesna Group	Standard Prophylaxis	Reference
1	1/169 (4%)	25/92 (27%)	Bremer et al. [25]
2	1/8 (12%)	7/8 (87%)	Bryant et al. [26]
3	44/1066 (4%)	312/409 (77%)	Scheef et al. [27]
4	7/67 (11%)	7/17 (41%)	Varini et al. [28]

[a] Mesna dosage was 20% of ifosfamide dose IV at 0, 4, and 8 hours.
[b] Standard prophylaxis includes hydration, diuretics, and alkalinization.
[c] Also includes bladder instillation of sulfhydryl compound.

mesna developed this finding ($p < 0.0001$). The ifosfamide dosage was also reduced solely for urotoxicity in 12 patients receiving NAC, while none of the patients receiving mesna required a dosage reduction because of urothelial toxicity. The different modes of administration of these two uroprotectants complicates the comparison. However, mesna given in this dosage and schedule provides better protection than orally administered NAC and allows better maintenance of drug dose [29].

Patients receiving cyclophosphamide in the usual dose of around 500–1000 mg/m^2 usually do not need urothelial prophylaxis, as the incidence of hematuria in this group of patients is low. However, higher dosages or a longer duration of cyclophosphamide administration is associated with a higher incidence of urotoxicity. Under this condition prophylactic measure may be required. Ifosfamide, with its different pharmacokinetic properties, is more urotoxic and hence is usually given with mesna. Another important use of mesna is in patients undergoing bone marrow transplantation who receive high-dose cyclophosphamide as a preparative regimen. Blacklock et al. reported that only 2 out of 20 transplant patients (10%) developed microhematuria [30]. They received 2400 mg/m^2 cyclophosphamide for 2 days. Link et al. also reported that only 1 out of 10 patients developed microhematuria with similar cyclophosphamide doses [31].

Patients with a history of hemorrhagic cystitis from prior cyclophosphamide or ifosfamide are also a difficult group of patients to treat. Mesna is effective in preventing further hematuria while retreating these patients with oxazaphosphorine. Andriole et al. [32] reported the retreatment of 26 patients with oxazaphosphorine-induced hematuria with mesna uroprotection. Seven patients with chronic hematuria received more therapy without worsening of their hematuria. Nineteen other patients with a previous history of hematuria received further therapy with ifosfamide or cyclophosphamide, and only two patients developed low-grade hematuria.

The usual recommended dosage of mesna given IV is 20% of the ifosfamide dose at the begining of ifosfamide therapy, repeating that dosage at 4 and 8 hours, and thus the total dosage is 60% of the total ifosfamide dose. At very high doses, the half-life of ifosfamide may be prolonged [10]. Patients receiving higher cyclophosphamide or ifosfamide doses probably would require a higher dose of mesna. The general recommendations are to give an extra dose at 12 hours or to increase the dose to 30% of the oxazaphosphorine dose. There are wide reported variations in the dosing of mesna, ranging from 60% to 160% of the oxazaphosphorine dose given over 8–12 hours every 3–4 hours. It has also been suggested that the urinary thiol concentration should be measured. This is impracticable in most routine situations. Even with an every 3- to 4-hour schedule, some patients do develop hematuria, as seen in table 1. This can happen if the patient passes urine before the next dose of mesna and no more mesna is present in the bladder to bind the oxazaphosphorine metabolites. One suggestion to overcome this problem is to give continuous-infusion mesna [23]. This might be particularly appropriate in patients receiving high doses or receiving concomitant nephrotoxic agents. The dose in this case is usually 10% of the oxazaphosphorine dose as an initial bolus and then 80–100% of the dose as continuous IV infusion over 24 hours. This type of administration would maintain a mesna level in the bladder throughout the oxazaphosphorine excretion. No clear data are available to prove the superiority of continuous infusion over every 4-hour boluses. Klein et al. showed that none of the 24 patients so treated by continuous infusion developed urotoxicity [33]. Of our 149 previously described, testicular cancer patients treated with ifosfamide and cisplatin and continuous-infusion mesna, only five (3.4%) developed urotoxicity [29].

A more convenient way to administer mesna would be oral administration. The recommended dose for oral mesna is an initial 20% of the oxazaphosphorine dose by IV bolus, followed by 40% of the oxazaphosphorine dose orally at 4 and 8 hours. The initial IV dose could also be administered as a 40% oral dose. Araujo et al. used oral mesna with 2250 mg/m^2 ifosfamide daily for 4 days in non-small-cell lung cancer patients. They reported 10 episodes of microscopic hematuria in 88 courses [34]. Oral mesna has a bad taste and administration is difficult and not recommended in patients who have problems with nausea and vomiting. It is also not recommended for higher dose oxazaphosphorine therapy. Oral mesna is still not commercially available in the United States.

Conclusion

In summary the urotoxicity from oxazaphosphorine could be successfully prevented by mesna. It is now routinely used in patients receiving oxazaphosphorine with the stated indications. With mesna urothelial toxicity no longer remains the dose-limiting toxicity, and it allows us to use these agents at higher dose. Amongst the variety of dosage schedules, the one preferred by us is continuous-infusion mesna at 100% of the total ifosfamide or a high-dose cyclophosphamide dose after initial 10% bolus dose. An acceptable alternative is mesna at 20% of the ifosfamide dose at 0, 4, and 8 hours. It will be important in the future to have more experience with the oral mesna preparation, which will make this therapy even easier to administer.

Acknowledgment

Supported in part by USPHS GCRC grant MOI-RROO 750-06.

References

1. Philips FS, Sternberg SS, Cronin AP, and Vidal PM. Cyclophosphamide and urinary bladder toxicity. Cancer Res 21:1577–1589, 1961.
2. Forni AM, Koss LG, and Geller W. Cytological study of the effect of cyclophosphamide on the epithelium of the urinary bladder in man. Cancer 171:1348–1355, 1964.
3. Jayalakshmamma B and Pinkel D. Urinary-bladder toxicity following pelvic irradiation and simultaneous cyclophosphamide therapy. Cancer 38:701–707, 1976.
4. Likes KE, Catchatourian R, Simon LS, and Gurwich, EL. Cyclophosphamide-induced hemorrhagic cystitis exacerbated by melphalan. Drug Int Clin Pharmacol 12:432–433, 1978.
5. Burkert H. Clinical overview of mesna. Cancer Treat Rev 10(Suppl. A):175–181, 1983.
6. Watson NA and Notley RB. Urologic complications of cyclophosphamide. Br J Urol 45:609, 1973.
7. Pyents RE, Droller MJ, and Bender WL. An approach to the control of massive hemorrhage in cyclophosphamide-induced cystitis by intravenous vasopressin. J Urol 120:253–254, 1978.
8. Brock N. Oxazaphosphorine cytostatics: past-present-future. Seventh Cain Memorial Award lecture (review). Cancer Res 49(1):1–7, 1989.
9. Brock N. The oxazaphosphorines. Cancer Treat Rev 10(Suppl. A):3–15, 1983.
10. Colvin M. The comparative pharmacology of cyclophosphamide and ifosfamide (review). Semin Oncol 9(Suppl. 1):2–7, 1982.
11. Brock N and Pohl J. The basis of modern ifosfamide therapy, introduction. In: Contri Oncol 26:1–11, 1987.
12. Brade WP, Merdrich K, and Varini M. Ifosfamide—pharmacology, safety and therapeutic potential. Cancer Treat Rev 12:1–47, 1985.
13. Hill DL. A review of cyclophosphamide. Charles C. Thomas, Springfield, IL, 1975.
14. Marti C, Steiner R, and Viollier AF. Systemic application of uromitexan to reduce urotoxicity. Contrib Oncol 5:57–59, 1981.
15. Morgan LR, Posey LE, Rainey J, Bickers J, Ryan D, Vial R, and Hull EW. Ifosfamide: a weekly dose fractionated schedule in bronchogenic carcinoma. Cancer Treat Rep 65:693–695, 1981.
16. Gad-El-Mawla N and Ziegler JL. Ifosfamide treatment of pancreatic cancer. Cancer Treat Rep 65(3–4):357–358, 1981.
17. Kovach JS, et al. A phase 2 study of intermittent high-dose isophosphamide therapy of advanced colorectal cancer. Oncology 29:34–39, 1974.
18. Ahmann DL, Hahn RG, and Bisel HF. A phase II evaluation of ifosfamide (NSC 109 724) treatment of disseminated breast cancer. Proc Am Assoc Cancer Res 15:1982, abstr. 794.

19. Scheef W, Klein HO, Burkert H, Gunther U, Hoefer-Janker H, Mitrenga D, Schnitker J, and Voigtmann R. Controlled clinical studies with an antidote against the urotoxicity of oxazaphosphorines: preliminary results. Cancer Treat Rep 63:501–505, 1979.
20. Brock N, Pohl J, and Stekar J. Studies on the urotoxicity of oxazaphosphorine cytostatics and its prevention. 2. Comparative study on the uroprotective efficacy of thiols and other sulfur compounds. Eur J Cancer Clin Oncol 17(11):1155–1163, 1981.
21. Pohl J. The toxicology, pharmacokinetics and interactions of uromitexan. In: Contrib Oncol 5:12–20, 1981.
22. Scheulen ME, Bremer K, Niederle N, Krischke W, Higi M, Seeber S, and Schmidt CG. Ifosfamide and etoposide in refractory testicular tumors. In: UICC Conference on Clinical Oncology, 1981. p. 129, abstr. 15-0373.
23. Shaw IC and Graham MI. Mesna—a short review. Cancer Treat Rev 14:47–86, 1987.
24. Shaw IC and Weeks MS. Excretion of disodium bis-2-mercaptoethanesulphonate (dimesna) in the urine of volunteers after oral dosing. Eur J Cancer Clin Oncol 23:933–935, 1987.
25. Bremer K, Scheulen ME, Niederle N, and Seeber S. Phase II evaluation of ifosfamide in refractory malignant diseases: comparison of the uroprotective effect of mesna with forced diuresis plus alkalinization of urine. In: Proc. 12th International Congress of Chemotherapy, Florence. Current Chemotherapy and Immunotherapy. ASM Publications, Washington, D.C., 1981, pp. 1394–1395.
26. Bryant BM, Jarman M, Ford HT, and Smith IE. Prevention of isophosphamide-induced urothelial toxicity with 2-mercaptoetehane sulphonate sodium (Mesnum) in patients with advanced carcinoma. Lancet 2:657–659, 1980.
27. Scheef W. Clinical experience with mesna (Uromitexan). In: 12th Int. Chemotherapy Congress Florenz, 1981, S.85.
28. Varini M, Ficarra G, and Monfardini S. Ifosfamide treatment with and without the uroprotective agent mesna. In: 12th International Congress of Chemotherapy, Florence, 1981, abstr. 176.
29. Munshi NC, Loehrer PJ, Williams SD, Langefeld C, Sledge G, Nichols CR, Roth B, Wassh W, Neumann A, and Einhorn LH. Comparison of N-acetylcysteine (NAC) and mesna as uroprotective agents in ifosfamide combination therapy (abstr). Proc Am Soc Clin Oncol 8:130, 1989.
30. Blacklock H, Ball L, Knight C, Schey S, and Prentice G. Experience with mesna in patients receiving allogeneic bone marrow transplants for poor prognostic leukemia. Cancer Treat Rev 10(Suppl. A):45–52, 1983.
31. Link H, Neef V, Niethammer D, and Wilms K. Prophylaxis of haemorrhagic cystitis due to cyclophosphamide-conditioning for bone marrow transplantation. Blut 43:329–330, 1981.
32. Andriole G, Sandlund JT, Miser JS, Arasi V, Linehan M, and Magrath IT. The efficacy of mesna (2-mercaptoethane sodium sulfonate as a uroprotectant in patients with hemorrhagic cystitis receiving further orazaphosphonic chemotherapy. J Clin Oncol 5:799–803, 1987.
33. Klein HA, Wickramanayake P, Dias, Coerper C, and Christian E. High-dose ifosfamide and mesna as continuous infusion over five days—a phase I/II trial. Cancer Treat Rev 10(Suppl A):167–173, 1983.
34. Araujo CE and Tessler J. Treatment of ifosfamide-induced urothelial toxicity by oral administration of sodium 2-mercaptoethane sulphonate (MESNA) to patients with inoperable lung cancer. Eur J Cancer Clin Oncol 19:195–201, 1983.

8. The role of progesterone receptors in meningioma

Steven M. Grunberg

Introduction

The recognition, description, and investigation of the role of hormone receptors, particularly progesterone receptors, in the growth of meningioma and the potential value of this information in the treatment of meningioma demonstrate a particularly rewarding interaction between the oncologist, the epidemiologist, the pathologist, the endocrinologist, and the neurosurgeon. Associations first described in case reports led to epidemiologic studies that confirmed these clinical impressions. Analysis of meningiomas by hormone receptor assay suggested a mechanism responsible for the clinical observations. These hormone receptor assays have recently been confirmed, in turn, by immunohistochemical studies. Appreciation of this mechanism has now resulted in clinical trials of hormonal manipulation for the control of unresectable meningioma.

Epidemiology

Meningiomas account for approximately 18% of intracranial neoplasms and are found most commonly in middle-aged women [1]. This predilection for female patients first brought attention to the possible role of female sex hormones in the growth of meningioma. Intracranial meningiomas are found approximately twice as often in women as men. However, the incidence for spinal meningioma increases to a 9:1 ratio in favor of female patients [2].

Since the report by Cushing [3] of spontaneous improvement of a meningioma after pregnancy, the relationship of meningioma to pregnancy has been a matter of interest. Although the incidence of meningioma among pregnant and nonpregnant women as a percentage of all brain tumors would appear to be similar, meningioma does show a tendency to become more symptomatic in the later stages (second and third trimester) of pregnancy [4]. Appreciation of the symptoms of meningioma is particularly important to the obstetrician, since early symptoms, such as nausea, may be considered to be related to the pregnancy itself, while later symptoms may be

Franco M. Muggia (ed.), NEW DRUGS, CONCEPTS AND RESULTS IN CANCER CHEMOTHERAPY.

Kluwer Academic Publishers, Boston. *ISBN 0-7923-1253-8*

initially viewed as suggestive of preeclampsia and may lead to a delay in diagnosis. Numerous authors [5–8] since Cushing have also noted the improvement in symptoms of meningioma after pregnancy. This waxing and waning pattern may lead to repeated episodes of worsening of symptoms during, and relief of symptoms after, successive pregnancies.

Changes in meningioma size have been documented by Michelsen [7], who obtained serial angiograms of a pregnant patient with a meningioma during and after her pregnancy, demonstrating the increase and decrease in displacement of the pericallosal artery. Controversy has arisen as to whether these changes are the result of hormone-related hyperplasia occurring during pregnancy or the result of cellular edema without hyperplasia related to increased vascularity and changes in the meningioma intercellular milieu during pregnancy. Weyand [5] described foamy swollen cytoplasm in two meningioma specimens removed from patients during pregnancy and suggested that these findings were consistent with the hypothesis of increased cellular edema. However, Goldberg [9] described removal of a cerebral meningioma from a pregnant patient in whom the meningioma tissue was estrogen receptor negative but progesterone receptor positive, and suggested that this finding might support a role for hormonal influence on the natural history of meningiomas. Benzel [10] has recently suggested a unifying mechanism for the roles of progesterone sensitivity and increased cellular edema in the natural history of meningioma by noting a statistically significant correlation between progesterone receptor positivity and computed tomography (CT) evidence of peritumoral edema ($p < 0.005$) in a series of 22 meningioma patients.

A third line of evidence suggesting a role for female sex hormones in meningioma growth is the observed association of meningioma with breast cancer [11–13]. Two epidemiologic studies have confirmed the anecdotal observations of this association. Schoenberg [14] used the records of the Connecticut Tumor Registry from 1935 to 1964 to identify patients with multiple primary tumors, at least one of which was within the central nervous system. The only significant correlation was that between breast cancer and meningioma (8 cases of meningioma observed compared to 3.37 cases expected, $p < 0.05$). Emry [15], using the Los Angeles County Tumor Registry, also identified a significant association between meningioma and breast cancer, but only when the diagnosis of meningoma followed that of breast cancer (37 observed cases versus 10.5 expected cases, $p < 0.001$).

Progesterone and estrogen receptors

The epidemiologic evidence suggesting a role for female sex hormones in the growth of meningioma led Donnell [16] to investigate the possibility of the presence of hormone receptors on meningioma. Donnell [16] assayed six meningioma specimens for the presence of estrogen receptor protein and did

Table 1. Estrogen and progesterone receptors in meningioma

Author	Estrogen Receptors Positive/Total (%)		Progesterone Receptors Positive/Total (%)		Reference
Donnel	4/6	(67)	—		16
Schnegg	0/10	(0)	4/10	(40)	17
Tilzer	0/6	(0)	4/6	(67)	18
Yu	15/16	(94)	9/11	(82)	19
Markwalder	20/34	(59)	26/34	(76)	20
Blankenstein	0/20	(0)	18/20	(90)	21
Vaquero	0/8	(0)	7/8	(87)	22
Pertuiset	43/60	(72)	62/64	(97)	23
Whittle	0/20	(0)	11/20	(55)	24
Martuza	25/42	(60)	16/22	(73)	25
Courriere	0/12	(0)	10/12	(83)	26
Reubi	5/13	(38)	11/13	(85)	27
Ironside	0/45	(0)	24/45	(53)	28
Grunberg	1/17	(6)	11/16	(69)	29
Puunonen	0/4	(0)	3/4	(75)	30
Whittle	0/29	(0)	16/29	(55)	31
Lesch	28/70	(40)	53/70	(76)	32
Benzel	0/22	(0)	19/22	(86)	10
Kornblum	1/29	(3)	8/29	(28)	33
Halper	1/49	(2)	37/49	(76)	34
Lee	6/17	(35)	14/17	(82)	35
Total	149/529	(28)	363/501	(72)	

indeed find significant amounts of estrogen receptor protein in 4 of 6 specimens. This study led to later studies by numerous authors [10, 17–35] in which both estrogen receptor protein and progesterone receptor protein were assayed. Although baseline values in different laboratories and under different assay conditions may differ, these later studies [10, 17, 18, 20–35] have consistently demonstrated a preponderance of progesterone receptor positivity over estrogen receptor positivity (table 1). On the whole the incidence of progesterone receptor positivity in meningioma is approximately 40% higher than that of estrogen receptor positivity. No correlation between progesterone receptor positivity and meningioma location has been described [20, 24, 31, 33]. Examination of progesterone receptor positivity compared to histologic type has suggested that anaplastic meningioma [32], and possibly fibrous meningioma [20], may have a lower incidence of progesterone receptor positivity.

The presence of progesterone or estrogen binding does not in itself demonstrate that a specific receptor protein exists. Schwartz [36] has suggested that the progesterone and estrogen binding proteins of meningioma may not meet the specificity criteria of true receptor proteins. Schwartz [36] reported significant competition for the progesterone binding sites of meningioma by estradiol, diethylstilbestrol, cortisol, dexamethasone, and dihydrotestosterone, while competition for estrogen binding sites was noted with progesterone, R5020, cortisol, and dihydrotestosterone. However, several other authors, including Markwalder [20], Blankenstein [21], and Ironside [28], have demonstrated high-grade specificity for the progesterone binding protein and have supported the hypothesis that this protein is indeed a classic progesterone receptor.

The classic model of a hormone-dependent tumor is that of breast cancer, in which binding of estrogen to estrogen receptors is the primary interaction and the generation of progesterone receptors depends upon the activity of estrogen receptors [37]. However, the dominance of a meningioma progesterone receptor independent of the estrogen receptor would not be a unique situation, since a parallel receptor situation can be found in the T47D breast cancer cell line in which an extremely high level of progesterone receptors generated independently of estrogen receptors is also seen [38].

Immunohistochemical identification of progesterone receptors

Further evidence for the existence of classic progesterone receptors but not classic estrogen receptors on meningiomas has recently been supplied through immunohistochemical staining methodology. Blankenstein [39], using a monoclonal antibody against the human estrogen receptor, was unable to detect specific staining in 21 meningioma specimens, 10 of which were considered to be estrogen receptor positive based on receptor assays with Scatchard analysis [40]. However, several authors [34, 41–43] have now demonstrated positive immunohistochemical staining of meningioma specimens using monoclonal antibodies against the human progesterone receptor. Press [41] and Waelti [42] demonstrated positive nuclear immunoreactivity for progesterone receptor in 2 of 4 meningioma specimens and 5 of 6 meningioma specimens, respectively. Blankenstein [43] showed an excellent correlation between Scatchard analysis [40] for progesterone receptor and progesterone receptor enzyme immunoassay using a monoclonal antibody in 24 meningioma specimens ($R = 0.9171$, $p < 0.001$). Halper [34] also noted a correlation between biochemical and immunohistochemical determinations of progesterone receptor positivity in 38 of 44 (86%) meningioma specimens assayed by both methodologies. The specificity of progesterone receptors in meningioma would, therefore, seem to have been well demonstrated, while the similarity of meningioma progesterone receptors and breast cancer progesterone receptors is strongly suggested by similar monoclonal antibody immunohistochemical staining.

Physiologic role of hormone receptors

The presence of progesterone receptors on meningiomas does not necessarily imply a functional role. In particular, the uncoupling of progesterone recep-

Table 2. Hormonal modulation of meningioma growth

Author	System	Hormonal Agents	Results	Reference
Jay	Cell culture	Estradiol Progesterone Tamoxifen	10–100% growth stimulation by estradiol in 4/4 meningiomas 10–44% growth stimulation by tamoxifen in 4/4 meningiomas 4–59% growth stimulation by progesterone in 4/4 meningiomas Antagonistic effect of estradiol + tamoxifen Antagonistic effect of estradiol + progesterone	44
Olson	Cell culture	Estradiol Progesterone Tamoxifen RU486	21–36% growth stimulation by estradiol in 3/3 meningiomas 25% growth stimulation by progesterone in 1/3 meningiomas 36% growth inhibition by progesterone in 1/3 meningiomas 19–35% growth stimulation by tamoxifen in 2/3 meningiomas 18–36% growth inhibition by RU486 in 3/3 meningiomas	45
Grunberg	Clonogenic assay	Estradiol Progesterone	Growth inhibition by estradiol in 2/13 meningiomas (0/1 estrogen receptor positive meningiomas) Growth inhibition by progesterone in 4/15 meningiomas (4/10 progesterone receptor positive meningiomas)	29
Maiuri	Cell culture	Estrogen Progesterone	No effect of estrogen Growth suppression by progesterone in 4/6 meningiomas Growth suppression by progesterone is not reversed by estrogen	46
Waelti	Cell culture	Medroxy-progesterone acetate	Growth inhibition in 6/17 meningiomas	47
Olson	Nude mouse	RU486	Disappearance of implanted meningioma nodules in 2/3 mice	50
Olson	Cell culture	Dihydro-testosterone	9–11% growth stimulation in 2/3 meningiomas	51
Reubi	Cell culture	SMS 201–995 (somatostatin analogue)	No change in incorporation of tritiated thymidine by 6 meningiomas	53
Kunert-Radek	Cell culture	Somatostatin	Significant decrease in incorporation of tritiated thymidine by 2 meningiomas	54

tor from estrogen receptor could imply that progesterone receptors had lost their physiologic significance and their ability to affect meningioma growth. However, a series of cell culture and animal studies do indeed suggest that hormonal modulation of meningioma growth is possible (table 2). Jay [44], using a cell culture model, demonstrated stimulation of meningioma growth in four cases by estradiol, tamoxifen, or progesterone. However, both tamoxifen and progesterone were antagonistic to estradiol when simultaneous exposure with estradiol was attempted. Olson [45], also using a celi culture system, demonstrated mild stimulation of meningioma growth by estradiol in 3 of 3 meningioma specimens, tamoxifen in 2 of 3 specimens, and progesterone in 1 of 3 specimens. However, progesterone also caused growth inhibition in 1 of 3 specimens in this study. Grunberg [29] examined the effects of estradiol and progesterone on meningioma growth using a human tumor stem-cell clonogenic assay. No definite effect of estradiol was demonstrated. However, 4 of 10 progesterone receptor positive meningioma specimens showed significant suppression of growth in the human tumor stem-cell clonogenic assay when exposed to progesterone. Maiuri [46], using a cell culture system, noted no effect of estrogen, but marked growth suppression by progesterone in 4 of 6 meningioma specimens. The progesterone effect was not reversed by the addition of estrogen. Waelti [47] noted growth inhibition of 6 of 17 meningioma specimens by medroxyprogesterone acetate in cell culture but could not correlate this growth inhibition with progesterone receptor content. Markwalder [48] compared meningioma specimens from eight patients pretreated with medroxyprogesterone acetate to specimens from five patients without pretreatment. In the specimens from pretreated patients, a significantly lower precentage of cells could be stained with Ki-67, a monoclonal antibody specific for proliferating cells.

Very exciting work on the effect of homonal modulation on meningioma growth has been performed using the progesterone antagonist RU486. RU486 is known to inhibit the growth of the progesterone receptor positive human breast cancer cell lines MCF7 and T47D [49]. Olson [45], using a cell culture system, demonstrated ihibition of meningioma growth by RU486 in 3 of 3 specimens. Olson [50] then examined the effect of RU486 on meningioma specimens implanted in nude mice and noted the disappearance of meningioma tumor nodules in 2 of 3 nude mice treated with RU486.

Other hormone receptors

Hormone receptors other than progesterone and estrogen receptors have been identified on meningioma specimens (table 3). Several groups have assayed meningiomas for the presence of androgen receptors. Schnegg [17] found androgen receptors on 2 of 9 meningioma specimens, while progesterone receptors were present on 4 of 10 specimens. No correlation between the presence of androgen receptors and progesterone receptors was noted.

Table 3. Androgen and somatostatin receptors in meningioma

Author	Androgen Receptors Positive/Total (%)	Somatostatin Receptors Positive/Total (%)	Reference
Schnegg	2/9 (22)	—	17
Pertuiset	23/25 (92)	—	23
Lesch	33/70 (47)	—	32
Kornblum	8/29 (28)	—	33
Lee	8/19 (42)	—	35
Olson	8/8 (100)	—	51
Reubi	—	50/50 (100)	52
Total	82/160 (51)	50/50 (100)	

Lee [35] found androgen receptors on 8 of 19 (42%) meningioma specimens and progesterone receptors on 14 of 17 (82%) meningioma specimens. Kornblum [33] detected both androgen and progesterone receptors on 8 of 29 (28%) meningioma specimens. Pertuiset [23] assayed meningioma cytosolic specimens and detected progesterone receptors in 43 of 46 (93%) specimens, androgen receptors in 23 of 25 (92%) specimens, and estrogen receptors in 14 of 46 (30%) specimens. In the largest reported series of meningiomas assayed for androgen receptors, Lesch [32] reported high levels of progesterone receptors on 53 of 70 (76%) meningoma specimens, moderate levels of androgen receptors on 33 of 70 (47%) meningioma specimens, and low levels of estrogen receptors on 36 of 70 (51%) meningioma specimens. Lesch [32] noted a correlation between the presence of estrogen receptors and androgen receptors, and between the presence of progesterone receptors and androgen receptors. Olson [51] detected low levels of androgen receptors in 8 of 8 meningioma specimens and performed cell culture growth assays on three of these specimens. A 10% stimulation of cell growth after 28 days exposure to dihydrotestosterone was demonstrated in 2 of 3 specimens, but was not considered to represent significant growth modulation.

Reubi [52] has now demonstrated specific somatostatin receptors on 50 human meningioma specimens. Although Reubi [53] did not note any effect of the somatostatin analogue SMS 201–995 on incorporation of tritiated thymidine by cell cultures from six meningioma specimens, Kunert-Radek [54] has reported a significant decrease in incorporation of tritiated thymidine by cell cultures from two meningioma specimens after exposure to somatostatin.

Clinical trials

A limited number of clinical trials attempting hormonal modulation of meningioma growth have been reported. Based on the initial reports of estrogen receptor positivity in meningiomas, Markwalder [55] initiated a trial of the antiestrogen tamoxifen administered for 8–12 months. A possible minor response was seen in 1 of 6 patients, but the use of antiestrogen therapy was not considered by the authors [55] to be promising. An explanation for the lack of effect of tamoxifen therapy on meningioma, in spite of the association of meningioma with breast cancer and the marked responsiveness of breast cancer to tamoxifen, has been suggested by Magdelenat [56]. Magdelenat [56] performed hormone receptor assays on meningioma and breast cancer specimens from the same patient and found the breast cancer specimen to be estrogen receptor positive/progesterone receptor negative, while the meningioma specimen was estrogen receptor negative/progesterone receptor positive. Although both tumors might indeed be hormone dependent, different therapeutic hormonal modulations would seem to be required. Markwalder [57] and Jaaskelainen [58] have investigated the use of medroxyprogesterone acetate, a progesterone agonist with efficacy against breast cancer, in the treatment of meningioma. Markwalder [57] demonstrated a marked reduction in measured progesterone receptor values of meningioma specimens in patients treated with medroxyprogesterone acetate prior to craniotomy compared to progesterone receptor values in a historical control series of meningiomas, suggesting that orally administered medroxyprogesterone acetate can indeed bind to meningioma. However, Jaaskelainen [58] treated five patients with unresectable meningioma with medroxyprogesterone acetate for periods ranging from 17 to 29 weeks and noted no clinical response. Grunberg [59] has reported the use of the progesterone agonist megestrol acetate in the treatment of nine patients with unresectable meningioma for periods from 1 to 12 months. No responses were noted, while three patients may have experienced acceleration of meningioma growth, as indicated by deterioration of vision. Grunberg [60] has recently reported minor objective regression of meningioma in 5 of 14 patients (accompanied in three cases by subjective improvement) following long-term treatment with the progesterone antagonist RU486.

Conclusion

Epidemiologic evidence suggesting a hormone dependence of meningioma, including the preponderance of meningiomas in female patients, the waxing and waning of meningioma-related symptoms with pregnancy, and the association of breast cancer with meningioma, led to the detection of hormone receptors on meningioma specimens. Unlike the situation with breast cancer, progesterone receptors are much more common than estrogen receptors in meningioma. In vitro studies of hormonal manipulations have suggested that treatment with an antiprogestational agent may be most effective in the treatment of meningioma. Clinical studies of estrogen antagonists and progesterone agonists have not been effective in modulating the growth of unresectable meningioma. However, clinical use of progesterone antagonists may allow modulation of the growth of this tumor. Development of this body of knowledge has resulted from significant and rewarding collaborations between the epidemiologist, the laboratory researcher, and the clinician.

References

1. Quest DO. Meningiomas: an update. Neurosurgery 3:219–225, 1978.
2. Kepes JJ. Meningiomas—Biology, Pathology, and Differential Diagnosis. Masson Publishing, New York, 1982, pp. 17–19.
3. Cushing H and Eisenhardt L. Meningiomas arising from the tuberculum sellae with the syndrome of primary optic atrophy and bitemporal field defects combined with a normal sella turcica in a middle-aged person. Arch Ophthalmol 1:1–41, 1929.
4. Roelvink NCA, Kamphorst W, van Alphen HAM, and Rao R. Pregnancy-related primary brain and spinal tumors. Arch Neurol 44:209–215, 1987.
5. Weyand RD, MacCarty CS, and Wilson RB. The effect of pregnancy on intracranial meningiomas occurring about the optic chiasm. Surg Clin North Am 31:1225–1233, 1951.
6. Bickerstaff ER, Small JM, and Guest IA. The relapsing course of certain meningiomas in relation to pregnancy and menstruation. Neurol Neurosurg Psych 21:89–91, 1958.
7. Michelsen JJ and New PFJ. Brain tumor and pregnancy. J Neurol Neurosurg Psych 32: 305–307, 1969.
8. Manganiello PD, Meltz RC, and Andros GJ. Probable parasellar meningioma in a pregnant woman. Obstet Gynecol 53:43S–46S, 1979.
9. Goldberg M and Rapport ZH: Neurosurgical, obstetric and endocrine aspects of meningioma during pregnancy. Isr J Med Sci 23:825–828, 1987.
10. Benzel EC and Gelder FB. Correlation between sex hormone binding and peritumoral edema in intracranial meningiomas. Neurosurgery 23:169–174, 1988.
11. Smith FP, Slavik M, and MacDonald JS. Association of breast cancer with meningioma. Report of two cases and review of the literature. Cancer 42:1992–1994, 1978.
12. Mehta D, Khatib R, and Patel S. Carcinoma of the breast and meningioma. Association and management. Cancer 51:1937–1940, 1983.
13. Miller RE. Breast cancer and meningioma. J Surg Oncol 31:182–183, 1986.
14. Schoenberg BS, Christine BW, and Wisnant JP. Nervous system neoplasms and primary malignancies of other sites. The unique association between meningiomas and breast cancer. Neurology 25:705–712, 1975.
15. Emry JK. The Association between Breast Cancer and Meningiomas. Master's thesis (Biometry), University of Southern California, Los Angeles, California, 1984.
16. Donnell MS, Meyer GA, and Donegan WL. Estrogen-receptor protein in intracranial meningiomas. J Neurosurg 50:499–502, 1979.
17. Schnegg J-F, Gomez F, LeMarchand-Beraud T, and de Tribolet N. Presence of sex steroid hormone receptors in meningioma tissue. Surg Neurol 15:415–418, 1981.
18. Tilzer LL, Plapp FV, Evans JP, Stone D, and Alward K. Steroid receptor proteins in human meningiomas. Cancer 49:633–636, 1982.
19. Yu Z-Y, Wrange O, Haglund B, Granholm L, and Gustafsson J-A. Estrogen and progestin receptors in intracranial meningiomas. J Steroid Biochem 16:451–456, 1982.
20. Markwalder T-M, Zava DT, Goldhirsch A, and Markwalder RV. Estrogen and progesterone receptors in meningiomas in relation to clinical and pathologic features. Surg Neurol 20:42–47, 1983.
21. Blankenstein MA, Blaauw G, Lamberts WJ, and Mulder E. Presence of progesterone receptors and absence of oestrogen receptors in human intracranial meningioma cytosols. Eur J Cancer Clin Oncol 19:363–370, 1983.

22. Vaquero J, Marcos ML, Martinez R, and Bravo G. Estrogen- and progesterone-receptor proteins in intracranial tumors. Surg Neurol 19:11–13, 1983.
23. Pertuiset BF, Moguilewsky M, Magdelenat H, Martin PM, Philibert D, and Poisson M. Sex steroid receptors in human meningioma and glioma. In: Progress in Cancer Research and Therapy, Vol. 31, F Bresciani, RJB King, ME Lippman, M Namer, J-P Raynaud (eds). Raven Press, New York, 1984, pp. 561–568.
24. Whittle IR, Foo MS, Besser M, and Vanderfield GK. Progesterone and oestrogen receptors in meningiomas: biochemical and clinicopathological considerations. Aust NZ J Surg 54:325–330, 1984.
25. Martuza RL, Miller DC, and MacLaughlin DT. Estrogen and progestin binding by cytosolic and nuclear fractions of human meningiomas. J Neurosurg 62:750–756, 1985.
26. Courriere P, Tremoulet M, Eche N, and Armand J-P. Hormonal steroid receptors in intracranial tumours and their relevance in hormone therapy. Eur J Cancer Clin Oncol 21:711–714, 1985.
27. Reubi JC, Maurer R, Klijn JGM, Stefanko SZ, Foekens JA, Blaauw G, Blankenstein MA, and Lamberts SWJ. High incidence of somatostatin receptors in human meningiomas: biochemical characterization. J Clin Endocrinol Metab 63:433–438, 1986.
28. Ironside JW, Battersby RDE, Dangerfield VJM, Parsons MA, Timperley WR, and Underwood JCE. Cryostat section assay of oestrogen and progesterone receptors in meningiomas: a clinicopathological study. J Clin Pathol 39:44–50, 1986.
29. Grunberg SM, Daniels AM, Muensch H, Daniels JR, Bernstein L, Kortes V, and Weiss MH. Correlation of meningioma hormone receptor status with hormone sensitivity in a tumor stem cell assay. J Neurosurg 66:405–408, 1987.
30. Punnonen R and Kuurne T. Estrogen and progestin receptors in intracranial tumors. Hormone Res 27:74–77, 1987.
31. Whittle IR, Hawkins RA, and Miller JD. Sex hormone receptors in intracranial tumors and normal brain. Eur J Surg Oncol 13:303–307, 1987.
32. Lesch K-P, Schott W, Engl H-G, Gross S, and Thierauf P. Gonadal steroid receptors in meningiomas. J Neurol 234:328–333, 1987.
33. Kornblum JA, Bay JW, and Gupta MK. Steroid receptors in human brain and spinal cord tumors. Neurosurgery 23:185–188, 1988.
34. Halper J, Colvard DS, Scheithauer BW, Jiang N-S, Press MF, Graham ML, Riehl E, Laws ER Jr., and Spelsberg TC. Estrogen and progesterone receptors in meningiomas: comparison of nuclear binding, dextran-coated charcoal, and immunoperoxidase staining assays. Neurosurgery 25:546–553, 1989.
35. Lee L-S, Chi C-W, Change T-J, Chou M-D, Liu H-C, and Liu T-Y. Steroid hormone receptors in meningiomas of Chinese patients. Neurosurgery 25:541–545, 1989.
36. Schwartz MR, Randolph RL, Cech DA, Rose JE, and Panko WB. Steroid hormone binding macromolecules in meningiomas. Failure to meet criteria of specific receptors. Cancer 53:922–927, 1984.
37. Horwitz KB, Koseki Y, and McGuire WL. Estrogen control of progesterone receptor in human breast cancer: role of estradiol and antiestrogen. Endocrinology 103:1742–1751, 1978.
38. Horwitz KB, Mockus MB, and Lessey BA. Variant T47D human breast cancer cells with high progesterone-receptor levels despite estrogen and antiestrogen resistance. Cell 28: 633–642, 1982.
39. Blankenstein MA, Berns PMJJ, Blaauw G, Mulder E, and Thijssen JHH. Search for estrogen receptors in human meningioma tissue sections with a monoclonal antibody against the human estrogen receptor. Cancer Res 46:4268s–4270s, 1986.
40. Scatchard G. The attractions of proteins for small molecules and ions. Ann NY Acad Sci 51:660–672, 1949.
41. Press MF and Greene GL. Localization of progesterone receptor with monoclonal antibodies to the human progestin receptor. Endocrinology 122:1165–1175, 1988.

42. Waelti ER and Markwalder T-M. Immunocytochemical evidence of progesterone receptors in human meningiomas. Surg Neurol 31:172–176, 1989.
43. Blankenstein MA, van der Meulen-Dijk C, and Thijssen JHH. Assay of oestrogen and progestin receptors in human meningioma cytosols using immunological methods. Clin Chim Acta 165:189–195, 1987.
44. Jay JR, MacLaughlin DT, Riley KR, and Martuza RL. Modulation of meningioma cell growth by sex steroid hormones in vitro. J Neurosurg 62:757–762, 1985.
45. Olson JJ, Beck DW, Schlechte J, and Loh P-M. Hormonal manipulation of meningiomas in vitro. J Neurosurg 65:99–107, 1986.
46. Maiuri F, Montagnani S, Gallicchio B, Carandente M, Lanza GG, and D'Andrea F. Oestrogen and progesterone sensitivity in cultured meningioma cells. Neurol Res 11:9–13, 1989.
47. Waelti ER and Markwalder T-M. Endocrine manipulation of meningiomas with medroxyprogesterone acetate. Effect of MPA on growth of primary meningioma cells in monolayer tissue culture. Surg Neurol 31:96–100, 1989.
48. Markwalder T-M, Gerber HA, Waelti E, Schaffner T, and Markwalder RV. Hormonotherapy of meningiomas with medroxyprogesterone acetate. Immunohistochemical demonstration of the effect of medroxyprogesterone acetate on growth fractions of meningioma cells using the monoclonal antibody Ki-67. Surg Neurol 30:97–101, 1988.
49. Bardon S, Vignon F, Chalbos D, and Rochefort H. RU486, a progestin and glucocorticoid antagonist, inhibits the growth of breast cancer cells via the progesterone receptor. Clin Endocrinol Metab 50:692–697, 1985.
50. Olson JJ, Beck DW, Schlechte JA, and Loh P-M. Effect of the antiprogesterone RU-38486 on meningioma implanted into nude mice. J Neurosurg 66:584–587, 1987.
51. Olson JJ, Beck DW, MacIndoe JW, and Loh P-M. Androgen receptors in meningiomas. Cancer 61:952–955, 1988.
52. Reubi JC. Identification of somatostatin receptors in human tumors. Triangle 27:179–188, 1988.
53. Reubi JC, Horisberger U, Lang W, Koper JW, Braakman R, and Lamberts SWJ. Coincidence of EGF receptors and somatostatin receptors in meningiomas but inverse, differentiation-dependent relationship in glial tumors. Am J Pathol 134:337–344, 1989.
54. Kunert-Radek J, Stepien H, Radek A, and Pawlikowski M. Somatostatin suppression of meningioma cell proliferation in vitro. Acta Neurol Scand 75:434–436, 1987.
55. Markwalder T-M, Seiler RW, and Zava DT. Antiestrogenic therapy of meningiomas—a pilot study. Surg Neurol 24:245–249, 1985.
56. Magdelenat H, Pertuiset BF, Poisson M, and Philippon J. Steroid receptor status difference in recurrent intracranial meningioma and breast cancer in the same patient. J Neurooncol 4:155–157, 1986.
57. Markwalder T-M, Waelti E, and Konig MP. Endocrine manipulation of meningiomas with medroxyprogesterone acetate. Effect of MPA on receptor status of meningioma cytosols. Surg Neurol 28:3–9, 1987.
58. Jaaskelainen J, Laasonen E, Karkkainen J, Haltia M, and Troupp H. Hormone treatment of meningiomas: lack of response to medroxyprogesterone acetate (MPA). A pilot study of five cases. Acta Neurochir 80:35–41, 1986.
59. Grunberg SM and Weiss MW. Lack of efficacy of megestrol acetate in the treatment of unresectable meningioma. J Neurooncol 8:61–65, 1990.
60. Grunberg SM, Weiss MH, Spitz IM, Ahmadi J, Sadun A, Russell CA, Lucci L, and Stevenson LL. Treatment of unresectable meningiomas with the anti-progestational agent mifepristone. J Neurosurg 74:861–866, 1991.

9. Combined chemotherapy and radiotherapy in small-cell lung cancer

Thierry Le Chevalier, Rodrigo Arriagada, and Maurice Tubiana

Introduction

Although known to be one of the most chemoresponsive and radiosensitive solid tumors in adult patients, small-cell lung carcinoma (SCLC) still has a particularly poor prognosis, with a 2-year survival not exceeding 10% in most series [1–4].

A variety of prognostic factors have been reported in many studies, mostly retrospective in nature, including clinical, biological, and radiological parameters [1,5–7]. Among these, the so-called limited or extensive character of the disease is probably the most reproducible prognostic factor in multivariate analyses. Nevertheless, it is well known that most patients present with occult distant metastases; this fact accounts for the small proportion of patients that can be successfully treated by surgery and/or radiotherapy.

Combination chemotherapy is largely accepted today as the treatment of choice in SCLC. The role of adjuvant thoracic radiotherapy in limited disease has been much debated. The reason for the controversy is whether it should be delivered or not and, if so, what timing and fractionation may be applicable.

We will present here the rationale for combining chemotherapy (CT) and radiotherapy (RT) in limited SCLC, and the clinical results obtained with different combination schedules.

Rationale for CT and RT combinations in limited SCLC

Recurrence after complete remission on the primary tumor site, i.e., lung and mediastinum, frequently occurs in patients with bulky tumors, in particular, when they have been treated by CT alone or when the radiation dose has been insufficient (below 40 Gy). A dose-response relationship of up to 45–50 Gy (with conventional fractions) is suggested in SCLC, and a dose of 55 Gy can reduce the local recurrence rate to below 40% [8]. This dose is necessary, even when induction CT is able to achieve a clinical complete remission, and it emphasizes the lack of effective criteria to assess the presence of residual tumor: More than 80% of thoracic failures are observed after CT alone in cases of so-called complete remissions [9].

Franco M. Muggia (ed.), NEW DRUGS, CONCEPTS AND RESULTS IN CANCER CHEMOTHERAPY.

Kluwer Academic Publishers, Boston. *ISBN 0-7923-1253-8*

A simple calculation can illustrate the respective roles of RT and CT in the control of a tumor. Let us consider a tumor of 100 g (nearly 10^{11} cells) in which 1% of the tumor cells are clonogenic (10^9 cells). If the radiosensitivity of the tumor is within the average range (D_{50} of the cells equal to 2 Gy), the tumor control dose (TCD) is approximately 60 Gy in 30 fractions. If CT has reduced the number of cells by half, which corresponds to a partial remission, the TCD is 58 Gy; it is still 54 Gy if 90% of the tumor cells have been killed with CT. It is only when CT has caused a clinical complete regression of the tumor (residual tumor mass less than 100 mg) that RT given to eradicate the remaining subclinical disease can be reduced to $20 \times D_{50}$ (40 Gy).

Although there are good theoretical reasons to combine CT and RT, the choice of the timing of both modalities is of crucial importance. At least three factors have to be taken into account to guide this choice: the toxic effects, tumor repopulation, and risks of development of chemoresistance and radioresistance.

Toxic effects on normal tissues

Toxic effects on normal tissues have always been the limiting factor in any therapeutic strategy that is meant to eradicate malignant disease. Indeed, combinations of CT and RT can produce severe and even life-threatening complications. These have been mainly observed in the tissues located within the irradiated volume; thus, it would seem safer to avoid the administration of drugs associated with an elective toxic effect on those tissues, such as bleomycin, when the lung is irradiated [10]. This is not always possible, however. For example, although doxorubicin is highly toxic when the mediastinum is irradiated [11], its use is nevertheless recommended in SCLC in view of its therapeutic efficacy.

Experimental studies have shown that the timing of the two treatment modalities generally has a strong influence on the normal tissue reactions but much less influence on the tumor [12–15]. Toxic effects are more intensive when drugs and radiation are administered concurrently or with short time intervals between administrations, yet tumor response appears to be much less enhanced by concurrent administration [13, 15]. Thus it seems safer to aim at avoiding an enhancement of the radiation response for both normal tissues and tumor. For most drugs and normal tissues, a toxicity independence of the two modalities can be obtained by inserting an interval of at least 7 days between their deliveries [16, 17].

Tumor repopulation

If both CT and RT have to be given sequentially and in full doses, the consequence of this long protraction can be a high level of tumor repopulation [12, 18, 19]. If CT is given prior to RT, increased repopulation between dose fractions can then lessen the effect of subsequent RT. On the other hand, if RT is delivered first, it delays the administration of CT and thus allows further growth of occult distant metastases. For example, if the tumor doubling time is 1 month, which is a realistic figure for SCLC, a delay of 2 months would permit the metastases to become four times larger [12]. This is why CT is generally given first; however, RT cannot be delayed for too long because CT often has only a limited effect on bulky tumors and can even elicit the development of radioresistance. Therefore RT is usually delivered out after two to four cycles of CT.

At this point in time, there is an acceleration in the rate of proliferation of the remaining viable cells. Thus if the pretreatment doubling time is 1 month, after a few cycles of CT the repopulation doubling time may be as short as 6 days. If a conservative estimate of 2 weeks is taken, then, after a 2-month interruption caused by the RT course, the occult metastases located outside the irradiated volume would be 16 times larger. Such a marked increase in size of the metastases would considerably lower the efficacy of CT.

In view of the uncertainty about the extent of repopulation, the shortest delay between CT and RT is advisable, and a compromise must be found between a short one, with the aim of limiting repopulation, and a long one required to avoid an interaction between drugs and radiation.

Chemoresistance and radioresistance

In patients treated with CT, the main source of failure is the emergence of chemoresistant cells. The rationale of multiple-drug CT is to combine drugs without cross-resistance and with independent toxicity to normal tissues. However, when many drugs with synergistic antitumor activity are used in combination, individual drug doses must be reduced in order to avoid cumulative toxicity. Some of the drugs can only be toxic to normal cells and have no significant additional activity on tumor cell kill. One should, therefore, avoid combining drugs that have a high probability of cross-resistance. Moreover, even with the best drug combinations, acquired drug resistance may occur, and this emphasizes the usefulness of combining other non-cross-resistant therapeutic agents, such as ionizing radiations.

For any drug, there may be a variety of biological mechanisms of acquired resistance. If these biological changes occur as isolated defects, in general, the level of resistance is relatively low. However, multiple modes of resistance can occur in the same cell, leading to a high level of resistance. Numerous agents that inhibit DNA synthesis, including most cytotoxic agents, can dramatically increase the frequency of gene amplification, which is one of the mechanisms associated with the development of resistance, particularly when treatment is prolonged [20].

The probability of development of drug-resistant cells is much greater for large tumors. Irradiation is logical for the local control of a tumor in particular when a) it is bulky, b) there is a great likelihood that chemoresistance will develop, or c) its regression is not rapid under CT.

However, the combination of CT and RT is based on the postulate that there is no cross-resistance between cytotoxic drugs and ionizing radiations. No increase in radioresistance has been observed in cell lines made resistant to doxorubicin [21–23]; thus, acquired drug resistance does not necessarily imply radiation resistance.

Although cross-resistance to CT and RT appears to be an infrequent event, it may occur. The likelihood of this rare event may be increased following sequential combination of both modalities. Hence the development of radioresistance due to prolonged drug administration is a possibility that should not be overlooked. Acquired radioresistance in human tumors might, indeed, be more frequent than previously assumed.

Early administration of both modalities might be the best way to overcome the development of resistance. This conclusion is consistent with that of the mathematical model constructed by Goldie and Coldman on the assumption that mutations to resistance arise spontaneously, independent of treatment [24].

Clinical randomized trials comparing CT alone versus CT + RT in limited SCLC

Chemotherapy and thoracic irradiation have been combined using several different schedules in SCLC. As CT is highly effective in achieving tumor regression but not a complete response, an adjuvant local treatment can improve the local control and potentially the cure rate, at least in patients with limited disease. As most patients present with initially bulky and inoperable tumors, in most cases RT appears to be the best local treatment in SCLC. The timing schedule between the two modalities can be concurrent, sequential, or alternating. Eight randomized studies comparing chemotherapy alone to combined radiotherapy and chemotherapy have been reported in the literature and are summarized in table 1 [4, 25–31].

The trials varied in the chemotherapeutic regimen: the dose and timing of thoracic radiation; whether or not prophylactic cranial irradiation was given; and whether thoracic irradiation was delivered to all patients, only to complete responders, to complete and partial responders, or to nonprogressing patients. Radiotherapy was delivered sequentially in four trials, concurrently in three, and alternatingly in one, and the total radiation dose to the primary tumor and mediastinum ranged from 35 up to 50 Gy.

Combined modality treatment increased the complete response rate in 3 out of 4 trials for which information is available, while local relapse was significantly reduced in 5 out of 7, and survival was prolonged in 5 out of 8.

Nevertheless, even if chest irradiation may improve long-term survival and local control, the 2-year survival rate remains poor. The toxicity of

Table 1. Randomized trials comparing CT Alone to CT + RT in limited SCLC

Trial	Number of Patients	Timing	MST (Months) CT/CT + RT	2-Year Survival (%) CT/CT + RT	p	Local Relapse (%) CT/CT + RT	p	Ref.
Fox	124	Seq	11/12	1.6/10	S	55/35	p = 0.05	25
Souhami	371	Seq	7.5/8	8/8	NS	32/28	N.S.	4
Kies	93	Seq	13	25	NS	90/56	p = 0.01	26
Creech	243	Seq	n.a.	n.a.	S(r)	n.a.	n.a.	27
Osterlind	145	Conc	12/10	13/8	NS	85/61	p = 0.005	28
Bunn	74	Conc	12/16	12/28	S	61/41	p < 0.001	29
Perry	399	Conc	10.5/12–13.4	8/15–25	S	47/19–17	p = 0.0002	30
Perez	291	Alt	11.5/14	19/28	S	52/36	p = 0.02	31

S = significant; NS = not significant; Seq = sequential; Conc = concurrent; Alt = alternating; MST = median survival time; n.a. = not available; (r) = CT responders.

these therapeutic schedules must be carefully evaluated, and the moderate benefit of the combined treatment in these randomized trials is counterbalanced by the increased toxicity in some of the schedules tested.

Rationale for alternating delivery of CT and RT

In order to reconcile the needs for early administration of both agents and for sequential delivery of each modality without a long interruption, an alternating treatment schedule in which CT and RT are interdigitated was designed and developed at the end of the 1970s [12, 16]. This approach has several advantages:

- It avoids the cumulative toxic effects resulting from the concurrent administration of drugs and irradiation. Alternating two different treatment modalities with minimal cross-toxicity allows more time for critical normal tissue to recover after each modality, and the delivery of full doses of CT and RT is then possible.
- It avoids a long gap in the CT delivery and shortens the time interval between both agents. Therefore, it limits the role of tumor repopulation, and treatment intensity can be increased in accordance with the concept of drug dose intensity.

This alternating regimen is consistent with the data reported by Looney et al. in their experimental model [32]; most of these data were obtained from an experimental tumor of the rat hepatoma 3924A, which is responsive to both radiation and cytotoxic drugs but cannot be cured by either modality when used alone. The sequential administration of 150 mg/kg of cyclophosphamide (CPM) every 11 days in four consecutive doses controlled tumor growth over 1 month, increased lifespan, but produced no or very few cures. The sequential delivery of a local irradiation at a dose of 15 Gy every 11 days to 10 rats produced only two complete regressions of tumor. Daily irradiation with 2.5 Gy, 6 days/week, up to a total dose of 90 Gy prevented tumor growth but obtained only one cure out of 10 animals.

An alternating administration of 15 Gy of radiation and 150 mg/kg of CPM at 11-day intervals produced a 56% cure rate. To determine the optimal timing of administration of both modalities, the same radiation dose of 15 Gy was given 15, 11, 7 or 4 days before or after CPM. The relative effectiveness of these timings was evaluated by tumor growth delay. Seven days was found to be the optimal interval. Shorter intervals increased the toxic effects, and longer ones reduced the effectiveness on the tumor.

The optimal dose per fraction was found to be 2.5 Gy. Toxicity was reduced when the dose per fraction was decreased from 15 to 3.7 Gy. Below 2.5 Gy, the effectiveness on the tumor was diminished and the probability of survival decreased.

Finally, it was reported that multiple daily fractions were more effective than a single daily dose, because the normal tissue recovered more rapidly

than the tumor. The best results were obtained with three courses of multiple fractionated irradiation, with CPM given 7 days after each of the three courses.

The clinical investigation was developed simultaneously but independently in our institute. The basic concept behind this new regimen was to maintain the CT schedule so that any reduction in its effectiveness would be avoided and to combine an agent without cross-resistance as early as possible. In this schedule, RT is delivered in split courses during the traditional rest weeks during which no CT is administered [16]. CT is initiated without any delay, and the interval between the successive cycles is, as usual, approximately 4 weeks. RT starts 1 week after completion of the second CT course and is continued for 10–14 days with 1-week rest between both modalities.

The Gustave-Roussy experience with limited SCLC

We started the first prospective phase II trial in May 1980 with three co-operating centers (GROP: C.H.I. Créteil, H. Antoine Béclère, and Chevilly-Larue). A total of 169 patients with limited SCLC were included in three consecutive trials until 1986 (protocols 002, 004, and 006). Patients had received no prior RT, no more than one course of CT, and had histologically proven SCLC. Staging investigations included chest X-ray, full blood count, chemistries, fiberoptic bronchoscopy, bone-marrow biopsy, bone scan, liver ultrasound or CT scan, and brain scan or CT scan. All patients were aged <70 years and their Karnofsky performance status (PS) was ≥40%.

The treatment schedule is shown in figure 1. The protocols were designed to deliver relatively high-dose radiotherapy in three courses, alternating with combination chemotherapy, in order to maximize both local control and long-term survival in patients with limited disease. The first protocol (002) was initiated in 1980 and was completed 18 months later. At that time, we observed relatively severe hematological toxicity and a local recurrence rate of 17% at 1 year. These observations led us to substitute cisplatinum for methotrexate and to increase the total dose of thoracic radiotherapy (protocol 004). In 1985, we increased the dose of VP 16213 and cisplatinum in the first two CT cycles and the dose of the third RT course (protocol 006). Radiotherapy was initially delivered in two courses of 15 Gy in six fractions over 10 days (002) or 20 Gy in eight fractions over 12 days (004, 006) using anterior and posterior fields; the target volume included all the initially visible tumor (with a 1.5 cm margin of normal lung tissue), as well as the mediastinum and both hilar and supraclavicular regions. A third course of RT was given using two anterior-posterior (002) or lateral and oblique (004, 006) fields, sparing the spinal cord and delivering 15 Gy in six fractions over 10 days (002 and 004) or 25 Gy in 10 fractions over 17 days (006) on the

CT ↓	RT ↙ ↘		CT ↓	RT ↙ ↘		CT ↓	RT ↙ ↘		CT ↓	Maintenance
29	41	56	63	75	90	97	109	119	132/175 days	

002

Doxorubicin: 40 mg/m^2 d1
VP 16213: 75 mg/m^2 d1, 2, 3
Cyclophosphamide: 300 mg/m^2 d3, 4, 5, 6
Methotrexate : 400 mg/m^2 d2 + folinic acid rescue

004

Doxorubicin: 40 mg/m^2 d1
VP 16213: 75 mg/m^2 d1, 2, 3
Cyclophosphamide: 300 mg/m^2 d3, 4, 5, 6
Cisplatinum: 100 mg/m^2 d2

006

Doxorubicin: 40 mg/m^2 d1
VP 16213: 100 mg/m^2 d1, 2, 3
(2 first cycles, then 75 mg/m^2 d1, 2, 3)
Cyclophosphamide: 300 mg/m^2 d2, 3, 4, 5
Cisplatinum: 120 mg/m^2 d2
(2 first cycles then 100 mg/m^2 d2)

Figure 1. Design of Gustave Roussy and GROP studies.

initial tumor and mediastinum. Prophylactic cranial irradiation (PCI) was given during the first course of thoracic RT in protocols 002 and 004 at a dose of 30 Gy in 10 fractions overe 14 days. In protocol 006, patients in complete remission (CR) were included in a randomized trial of PCI at the end of the induction protocol (1 out of 2 did not receive PCI).

Patients in CR were given maintenance chemotherapy consisting of eight and six CT cycles, respectively, in protocols 002 and 004 [33]. Patients in 006 did not receive maintenance CT.

Four patients included in protocol 004, who were in complete remission after induction therapy, received intensive CT with autologous bone marrow transplantation as consolidation treatment, instead of maintenance CT. They have been reported elsewhere [34].

All patients were restaged following the sixth cycle of induction CT. Restaging was identical to the initial assessment. Criteria for tumor response and treatment toxicity were registered according to the WHO recommendations [35]. Chest X-ray was regularly performed, and any minor change was further investigated by fiberoptic bronchoscopy, in addition to those planned in the protocol. Prognostic factors were analyzed by a multiple regression model, as described by Cox [36].

Our population is presented in table 2. It consisted of 141 men and 28 women, and the mean age was 54 years. Mean PS according to the Karnofsky index was 85% (range 40–100%). Protocols 002 and 004 were pooled, as there was no difference in the population characteristics and results.

The results are presented in table 3. Local recurrence after complete remission was observed in 23% of patients in protocol 002 and 004, and in 12% of patients in protocol 006. Hematological toxicity was observed in all patients, and it occurred more frequently after the fourth chemotherapy course. Currently, 20 patients with a follow-up of more than 4 years are alive. The mean performance status (PS) of these long-term survivors is 85%.

Prognostic factors were studied in protocols 002 and 004. They were separately analyzed because of the differences in induction therapy (methotrexate versus cisplatinum and 45 Gy versus 55 Gy delivered to the tumor and mediastinum).

Table 2. Population: Limited SCLC. Gustave-Roussy and GROP studies

	Protocols 002 + 004	Protocol 006
Number of patients	109	60
Sex (M/F)	96/13	45/15
Mean age (years)	54	54
P.S. (Karnofsky index)	82%	85%
Stage (I–II/III)	10/99	10/50

Table 3. Results: Limited SCLC Gustave-Roussy and GROP studies

	Protocols 002 + 004	Protocol 006
Complete response rate	79%	72%
Median survival	17 mo.	16.5 mo.
Lethal toxicity	8%	12%
12-mo. overall survival	74%	71%
24-mo. overall survival	31%	35%
2-yr disease-free survival	27%	21%
4-yr disease-free survival	20%	—

Age, sex, T category, PS, drug doses/m^2 actually administered during the first course of chemotherapy, mean dose per course, and initial hematological toxicity were analyzed in order to determine their prognostic incidence in these trials.

The major prognostic factor was hematological toxicity of the first course of CT ($p < 0.03$) in protocol 002 [37], while it was the actual delivered dose of cyclophosphamide ($p < 0.001$) and cisplatin ($p < 0.002$) during the first course of CT in protocol 004 [38].

Our studies have proven the feasibility of these three protocols, provided that there is a very good coordination between involved oncologists. Tolerance appears to be acceptable, and our retrospective analysis of prognostic factors led us to initiate a randomized trial in order to determine the prognostic impact of the intensity of the first course of chemotherapy.

Treatment toxicity of combined CT and RT

Combination of CT and RT results in a critical increase in toxicities of both modalities, which is the major problem encountered with this therapeutic approach. The toxicities described for radiotherapy are increased, as CT is an active radiosensitizer. Similarly, in irradiated normal tissues, RT enhances the toxic effects of CT. The type of combination (concurrent, sequential, or alternating), the delay between CT and RT, the cytotoxic drugs used, the size of the fields, and the fractionation and dose of RT all intervene in the toxicity observed in the heterogeneous population of lung cancer patients treated with a combined approach.

Acute toxicity is particularly critical when CT and RT are given concurrently, as described in the randomized NCI study [29]. In this trial, the CT induction regimen included cyclophosphamide, methotrexate, and lomustine, and RT was delivered simultaneously in randomized patients. The nadir leukocyte counts were significantly lower and infections were greater in the CT-RT group than in the group receiving CT alone. Esophagitis occurred in 64% of patients and weight loss was significantly greater in the CT-RT group. However, no difference was observed in early mortality between the group receiving CT alone and the group treated with concurrent CT and RT.

Acute toxicity is apparently lower when CT and RT are given alternatively: In the SCSG study, when the combination of doxorubicin, cyclophosphamide, and vincristine were alternated with three RT courses, there was no significant increased toxicity for the combined modality group when compared with the patients treated with CT alone [31]. The tolerance of the Gustave-Roussy Institute alternating schedule is also acceptable when CT and RT are given with a 7-day interval between each modality [39].

A major problem with the combined RT and CT approach is the long-term toxicity. Long-term sequelae may occur in all irradiated organs (lung, esophagus, heart and pericardium, brain). In the NCI study, severe late pulmonary toxicity occurred in 21% of patients receiving concurrent CT and RT, and in 4% of patients receiving CT alone [29]; congestive heart failure developed in four patients treated with concurrent RT and CT, but only one in the CT group; five patients died of these toxicities in the combined therapy group versus two in the group treated with CT alone. On the other hand, severe or life-threatening toxicity was reported in only 1% of the patients in the SECSG study [31]. In our study, we investigated the pulmonary status of the first 18 patients who survived free of disease for more than 30 months after the initiation of treatment [40]. Exertional dyspnea was observed in eight patients (44%) and was disabling in two patients with previously symptomatic chronic obstructive lung disease (COLD). Endoscopic examination revealed sequelae in 65% (mainly cicatricial stenosis, mucosal vessel dilatation, and localized abnormal secretions). Pulmonary functional tests demonstrated nearly normal arterial blood gases, both at rest and after exercise, and a mild obstructive ventilatory defect in most patients (total pulmonary capacity, 88 $\pm$ 12; vital capacity, 72 $\pm$ 12; forced expiratory volume in 1 second, 69 $\pm$ 25; results expressed as % predicted values). RT-induced lung fibrosis was present on all chest X-rays and, after semiquantitative assessment, was found to be related only to the volume of irradiated lung ($p < 0.05$) and to the cumulative dose/m^2 of VP 16 received during the six CT cycles ($p < 0.01$, variance analysis), with no difference in patients treated with methotrexate or cisplatinum. Hence our results show that this late pulmonary toxicity is usually mild, but may lead to disabling respiratory impairment in patients with symptomatic COLD.

An important adverse effect of the combined treatment is the toxicity to the central nervous system. This has been widely reported, and implication in its causation has been the concurrent administration of systemic CT and brain RT and use of neurotoxic drugs. The importance of fractionation and the dose of RT have also been emphasized [41]. The degree of injury is variable, from asymptomatic CT scan abnormalities to dementia. The problem remains major in a population at high risk of developing brain metastases where prophylactic cranial irradiation has an undeniable effect on the prevention of brain metastases. Intensity and frequency of neurologic sequelae after prophylactic cranial irradiation depend on the quality of evaluations, and it is clear that the ongoing randomized trials in patients with SCLC in CR will provide valuable information.

Another aspect of long-term toxicity in our population concerns general conditions. Combined modality treatment is a deliberately aggressive approach, as we know that it is the only way to obtain more than 15% long-term survivors in limited SCLC. Even if a good proportion of long-term survivors do not exhibit symptomatic sequelae, we know that patients are rarely able to resume their previous lifestyle and that most of them will not return to work [41].

Finally a major complication that must be emphasized is the development of second malignancies, and particularly leukemia or preleukemia, as they are one of the risks of an aggressive treatment. It is difficult to evaluate the risk of secondary leukemia or preleukemia in long-term survivors, as such patients are relatively rare. Nevertheless, there is no doubt that the combined modality approach increases the risk of secondary acute nonlymphocytic leukemia, as reported in other malignancies, such as Hodgkin's disease [42]. Comparatively, the risk of secondary solid tumors does not appear to be increased, except for secondary NSCLC after SCLC [41]. In our experience, only one patient developed a second malignancy (cervical carcinoma).

Conclusions

Today, CT is the standard treatment for SCLC. However, when disease appears clinically limited to the thorax, the combination of CT and RT will yield a moderate but significant survival benefit compared to CT alone, as reported in the majority of randomized trials. New approaches in timing and fractionation of RT and CT recently reported [39, 43] have given promising results after an alternating or concurrent combination, but these encouraging results have yet to be confirmed in large randomized studies.

Alternating combination of CT and RT have also produced improved survival rates in some other malignant diseases, such as high-grade non-Hodgkin's lymphomas, but not in all. This emphasizes that there is not an ideal regimen effective in all types of malignancies [8, 12]. The choice of the combination regimen should take into account the biological characteristics of the tumors, as well as the specific toxicities associated with the drugs used in the treatment.

Acknowledgments

The authors thank Mrs. Lorna SAINT-ANGE and Mrs. Catherine LOGE for their help in preparing the manuscript.

References

1. Davis S, Wright PW, Schulman SF, Scholes D, Thorning D, and Hammar S. Long-term survival in small cell carcinoma of the lung: a population experience. J Clin Oncol 3:80–91, 1985.
2. Hansen M, Hansen HH, and Dombernowsky P. Long-term survival in small cell carcinoma of the lung. JAMA 244:247–250, 1980.
3. Lee JS, Unsawasdi T, Lee Y, Barkley HT, Murphy WK, Welch S, and Valdivieso M. Neurotoxicity in long-term survivors of small cell lung cancer. Int J Radiat Oncol Biol Phys 12:313–321, 1984.
4. Souhami RL, Geddes DM, Spiro SG, Harper PG, Tobias JS, Mantell BS, Fearon F, and Bradbury I. Radiotherapy in small cell cancer of the lung treated with combination chemotherapy: a controlled trial. Br Med J 288:1643–1646, 1984.
5. Maurer LH and Pajak TF. Prognostic factors in small cell carcinoma of the lung: a Cancer and Leukemia Group B study. Cancer Treat Rep 65:767–774, 1981.
6. Harper PG, Souhami RL, Spiro SG, Geddes DM, Guimaraes M, Fearon F, and Smyth JF. Tumor size, response rate and prognosis in small cell carcinoma of the bronchus treated by combination chemotherapy. Cancer Treat Rep 66:463–470, 1982.
7. Osterlind K, Hansen HH, Hansen M, Dombernowsky P, and Andersen PK. Long-term disease-free survival in small-cell carcinoma of the lung: a study of clinical determinants. J Clin Oncol 4:1307–1313, 1986.
8. Tubiana M, Arriagada R, Carde P, Cosset JM, and Le Chevalier T. Adjuvant radiotherapy in chemosensitive tumors. In: Adjuvant Therapy of Cancer V, SE Salmon (ed). Grune & Stratton, Orlando, pp. 25–34.
9. Choi NC, Propert K, Carey RW, Eaton W, Leone LA, Silberfarb P, and Green M. Accelerated radiotherapy followed by chemotherapy for locally recurrent small-cell carcinoma of the lung. A phase II study of Cancer and Leukemia Group B. Int J Radiat Oncol Biol Phys 13:263–266, 1987.
10. Rubin P. Late effects of chemotherapy and radiation therapy: a new hypothesis. Int J Radiat Oncol Biol Phys 19:5–34, 1984.
11. Lagrange JL, Thyss A, Caldani C, Hery M, Schneider M, and Bensadoun JR. Toxicity of combination of ABVD chemotherapy and mediastinal irradiation for Hodgkin disease patients with massive initial mediastinal involvement. Bull Cancer 75:801–806, 1988.
12. Tubiana M, Arriagada R, and Cosset JM. Sequencing of drugs and radiation. Cancer 55:2131–2139, 1985.
13. Fu KK. Biological basis for the interaction of chemotherapeutic agents and radiation therapy. Cancer 55:2123–2130, 1985.
14. Von Der Maase H. Experimental studies on interactions of radiation and cancer chemotherapeutic drugs in normal tissues and a solid tumor. Radiother Oncol 7:47–68, 1986.
15. Steel GC. The search for therapeutic gain in the combination of radiotherapy and chemotherapy. Radiother Oncol 11:31–53, 1988.
16. Tubiana M. Les associations radiothérapie-chimiothérapie. Bull Cancer 68:109–115, 1981.
17. Looney WB and Hopkins HA. Alternation of chemotherapy and radiotherapy in cancer management. III. Results in experimental solid tumors systems and their relationship to clinical studies. Cancer Treat Rep 70:141–162, 1986.
18. Tubiana M. Repopulation in human tumors. A biological background for fractionation in radiotherapy. Acta Oncol 27:83–88, 1988.
19. Withers HR, Taylor JMG, and Maciejewski B. The hazard of accelerated tumor clonogen repopulation during radiotherapy. Acta Oncol 27:131–146, 1988.
20. Schimke RT. Methotrexate resistance and gene amplification. Mechanisms and implications. In: Accomplishments in Cancer Research, JG Fortner and JE Rhoads (eds), JB Lippincott, Philadelphia, 1986, pp. 75.
21. Louie KG, Behrens BC, Kinsella TJ, Hamilton TC, Grotzinger KR, McKoy WM, Winker

MA, and Ozols RF. Radiation survival parameters of antineoplastic drug-sensitive and resistant human ovarian cancer cell lines and their modification by buthionine. Cancer Res 45:2110–2115, 1985.

22. Mitchell JB, Gamson J, Russo A, Friedman N, Degraff W, Carmichael J, and Glatstein E. Chinese hamster pleiotropic multidrug resistant cells are not radioresistant. NCI Monogr 6:187–191, 1988.
23. Wallner K and Li GC. Adriamycin resistance, heat resistance and radiation response in Chinese hamster fibroblasts. Int J Rad Oncol Biol Phys 12:829–833, 1986.
24. Goldie GH and Coldman AG. The genetic origin of drug resistance in neoplasm: implications for systemic therapy. Cancer Res 44:3643–3663, 1984.
25. Fox RM, Woods RL, Brodie GN, and Tattersall MHN. A randomized study: small cell anaplastic lung cancer treated by combination chemotherapy and adjuvant radiotherapy. Int J Rad Oncol Biol Phys 6:1083–1085, 1980.
26. Kies MS, Mira JG, Crowley JJ, Chen TT, Pazdur R, Grozea PN, Rivkin SE, Coltman CA, Ward JH, and Livingston RB. Multimodal therapy for limited small cell lung cancer: a randomized study of induction combination chemotherapy with or without thoracic radiation in complete responders; and with wide field versus reduced field radiation in partial responders: a Southwest Oncology Group study. J Clin Oncol 5:592–600, 1987.
27. Creech R, Richter M, and Finkelstein D, for the ECOG. Combination chemotherapy with or without consolidation radiation therapy (RT) for regional small cell carcinoma of the lung. Proc Am Soc Clin Oncol, abstract 756, 1988.
28. Osterlind K, Hansen HH, Hansen HS, Dombernovsky P, Hansen M, and Rorth M. Chemotherapy versus chemotherapy plus irradiation in limited small cell lung cancer: results of a controlled trial with 5 years' follow-up. Br J Cancer 54:7–17, 1986.
29. Bunn PA, Lichter AS, Makuch RW, Cohen MH, Veach SR, Matthews MJ, Johnston-Anderson A, Edison M, Glatstein E, Minna JD, and Ihde DC. Chemotherapy alone or chemotherapy with chest radiation therapy in limited stage small cell lung cancer: a prospective randomized trial. Ann Intern Med 106:655–662, 1987.
30. Perry MC, Eaton WL, Propert KJ, Ware JH, Zimmer B, Chahinian AP, Skarin A, Carey RW, Kreisman H, Faulkner C, Comis R, and Green MR. Chemotherapy with or without radiation therapy in limited small cell carcinoma of the lung. N Engl J Med 316:912–918, 1987.
31. Perez CA, Einhorn L, Oldham RK, Greco FA, Cohen HJ, Silerman H, Krauss S, Hornback N, Comas F, Omura G, Salter M, Keller JW, McLaren J, Kellermeyer R, Storaasli J, Birch R, and Dandy M. Randomized trial of radiotherapy to the thorax in limited small cell a preliminary report. J Clin Oncol 2:1200–1208, 1984.
32. Looney WB, Special lecture: alternating chemotherapy and radiotherapy. NCI Monogr 6:85–94, 1988.
33. Arriagada R, Le Chevalier T, Baldeyrou P, Pico JL, Ruffie P, Martin M, El Bakry HM, Duroux P, Bignon J, Lenfant B, Hayat M, Rouesse JG, Sancho-Garnier H, and Tubiana M. Alternating radiotherapy and chemotherapy schedules in small cell lung cancer, limited disease. Int J Rad Oncol Biol Phys 11:1461–1467, 1985.
34. Pico JL, Le Chevalier T, Baume D, Arriagada R, Beaujan F, and Hayat M. Phase I–II study of high dose chemotherapy (HDC) followed by autologous bone marrow transplantation (ABMT) in small cell lung cancer. European Society for Medical Oncology. Nice, November 28–30, 1986, abstract no. 225, 1986.
35. World Health Organization. Handbook for Reporting the Results of Cancer Treatment. WHO Offset, Publ. no. 48. World Health Organization, Geneva.
36. Cox DR. Regression models and life tables. J R Stat Soc 34:187–220, 1972.
37. Le Chevalier T, Arriagada R, De The H, De Cremoux H, Sancho-Garnier H, and Rouesse J. Toxicity of first chemotherapy cycle as major prognostic factor in survival of patients with limited small cell lung cancer (LSCLC). Proc Am Soc Clin Oncol 5:181, 1986.
38. Arriagada R, De The H, Thomas F, Ruffie P, De Cremoux H, Martin M, Duroux P,

Dewar J, Sancho-Garnier H, and Le Chevalier T. Limited small cell lung cancer: a possible prognostic impact of initial chemotherapy doses. Bull Cancer 76:605–615, 1989.

39. Le Chevalier T, Arriagada R, De The H, De Cremoux H, Martin M, Baldeyrou P, Ruffie P, Benna F, Cerrina ML, Sancho-Garnier H, and Hayat M. Combination of chemotherapy and radiotherapy in limited small cel lung carcinoma: results of alternating schedule in 109 patients. NCI Monogr 6:335–338, 1988.
40. De Cremoux H, Baldeyrou P, Martin M, Ruffie P, Arriagada R, and Le Chevalier T. Late pulmonary toxicity of alternating radiotherapy (RT) and chemotherapy (CT) in limited small cell lung cancer (SCLC). Role of VP 16. Proc Am Soc Clin Oncol, abstract 709, 1987.
41. Johnson BE, Ihde DC, Bunn PA, Becker B, Walsh T, Weinstein ZR, Matthews MJ, Whang-Peng J, Makuch RW, Johnston-Early A, Lichter AS, Carney DN, Cohen MH, Glatstein E, and Minna JD. Patients with small-cell lung cancer treated with combination chemotherapy with or without irradiation. Ann Intern Med 103:430–438, 1985.
42. Henry-Amar M. Quantitative risk of second cancer in patients in first complete remission for early stages of Hodgkin's disease. NCI Monogr 6:65–72, 1988.
43. Turrisi AT, Glover DJ, and Mason BA. Concurrent twice-daily radiotherapy plus platinum-etoposide chemotherapy for the treatment of limited small cell lung cancer: a preliminary report. In: Treatments Modalities in Lung Cancer, Antibiotics and Chemotherapy, Vol. 41, R Arriagada, and T Le Chevalier (eds). S. Karger, Basel, 1988, pp. 109–114.

Addendum to Chapter 2

Rakesh Goel and Stephen B. Howell

Interactions between dipyridamole and chemotherapeutic agents has greatly expanded recently.

Dipyridamole has been shown to potentiate the activity of several additional chemotherapy drugs in vitro, including actinomycin D [80, 81], daunorubicin [80, 81], mitoxantrone [82], teniposide (VM-26) [80], melphalan [80], and 10-ethyl-10-deasaaminopterin (10-EDAM) [83]. Several researchers have observed that the modulation of chemotherapeutic agents by dipyridamole takes place in vivo [84–87]. Keane et al. showed that dipyridamole significantly potentiated the cytotoxicity of cisplatin against both transplanted human bladder carcinoma and human embryonal germ cell carcinoma in nude mice without any significant increase in host toxicity [84]. They later compared the comparative ability of dipyridamole to affect the therapeutic index of cisplatin, carboplatin, and etoposide in athymic nude mice carrying transplanted bladder carcinoma [85]. They concluded that an enhanced therapeutic index was maximal with cisplatin, low with carboplatin, and almost non-existent with etoposide. Sakaguchi et al. observed that dipyridamole significantly potentiated doxorubicin's ability to inhibit the appearance of lung metastases in mice injected with B16 melanoma cells intravenously [86]. Cao et al. showed that the combination of dipyridamole and amphotericin B significantly potentiated the inhibitory effect of 5-fluorouracil or methotrexate against a panel of transplantable tumors in mice including sarcoma 180, cervical carcinoma U14, and Lewis lung carcinoma, without any significant increase in host toxicity [87].

At this point in time, the synergy between dipyridamole and anticancer drugs has not yet been definitely demonstrated in humans, although the preliminary data is encouraging [32, 34–38, 47–53, 55, 62, 65, 88]. However, we have studied the in vivo biologic activity of the dipyridamole in the peritoneal fluid of patients who received a continuous infusion of intraperitoneal methotrexate and dipyridamole [39, 89]. We found that the uptake of [^{3}H]-uridine in OV 2008 cells incubated in aliquots of peritoneal fluid in which steady-state concentrations of dipyridamole and methotrexate had been achieved, was reduced to a mean of 16% ± 11% (SD) of control. Thus, the bioassay corroborated that the concentrations of biologically active dipyridamole achieved in the peritoneal fluid of patients entered into this study were sufficient to produce biochemical modulation of methotrexate via its ability to inhibit cellular nucleoside uptake [89].

Potentiation of the activity of chemotherapy drugs in multidrug-resistant cells has also been studied. Asoh et al. showed that dipyridamole increased the cytotoxicity of both vincristine and actinomycin D in the VJ-300 and HC-7-5-/VCR cell lines (which are multidrug-resistant (mdr) variants of human cancer KB and HC-7-5 cell lines respectively) [80]. The efflux of both drugs (but not of doxorubicin or daunomycin) was significantly decreased in both mdr cell lines. Dipyridamole also increased the cellular uptake by 1.5- to 2-fold of both drugs in the two mdr cell lines. Dipyridamole and verapamil both inhibited photoaffinity labeling with [^{3}-H]azidopine of P-glycoprotein in VJ-300 cells.

Shalinsky et al. studied the ability of dipyridamole to enhance the drug sensitivity to etoposide, vinblastine, and colchicine using the drug-sensitive epidermoid line KB-3-1 and two drug-resistant variants, KB-GRC1 and KBV1 cell lines (the latter two cell lines both expressing P-glycoprotein) [90]. They also studied the interaction of dipyridamole with vinblastine in parenteral HT080 cells and a multidrug-resistant variant, DR4, which lacks mdrl expression [91]. They showed that dipyridamole can produce synergy independently of mdrl expression but much greater levels of synergy are achievable in mdrl-expressing tumor cells. Both groups of investigators felt that dipyridamole can potentiate the action of chemotherapy drugs in multidrug-resistant cells by P-glycoprotein-independent and -dependent mechanisms [80,90,91].

Strategies to overcome drug resistance clinically have recently included dipyridamole [88]. They conducted a phase I study aiming to selectively increase the sensitivity of etoposide to tumors confined to the peritoneal cavity. Both drugs were administered as a continuous 72-hour infusion to 16 patients. The maximum tolerated daily dose of etoposide was 175 mg/m^2 with a fixed daily dose of $24/m^2$ dipyridamole. The dose-limiting toxicities were leukopenia and thrombocytopenia. The free dipyridamole and etoposide concentrations achieved in the peritoneal cavity were within the ranges that were needed for the synergistic interaction of the two drugs in vitro [70,71,90,91].

Bibliography

80. Asoh K, Saburi Y, Sato S, Nogae I, Kohno K, and Kuwano M. Potentiation of some anticancer agents by dipyridamole against drug-sensitive and drug-resistant cancer cell lines. Jap J Cancer Res 80:475–481, 1989.
81. Kusumoto H, Maehara Y, Sakaguchi Y, Kohnoe S, Kumashiro R, and Sugimachi K. Modulation of cytotoxic effect of anticancer drugs by dipyridamole in HeLa cells in vitro. Anticancer Res 10:1643–1645, 1990.
82. Desai PB, and Sridhar R. Effect of chemical modifiers on the toxicity of mitoxantrone towards CHO-K cells in vitro. Proc Am Assoc Cancer Res 30:559, 1989.
83. Dearing MP, Englee-Miller MJ, Kramer BS, Chou E, Mulshine JL, and Gadzar AF. Enhanced cell kill of human lung cancer cell lines by 10-Ethyl-10-deazaaminopterin (10-EDAM) when given with Dipyridamole (DPM). Proc Am Assoc Cancer Res 31:17, 1990.
84. Keane TE, Rosner G, Donaldson JT, Norwood DL, Poulton SH, and Walther PJ. Dipyridamole-cisplatin potentiation: enhanced in vivo cytotoxicity in xenograft models of human testicular and bladder cancers. J Urology 144:1004–1009, 1990.
85. Gingrich JR, Keane TE, and Walther PJ. Disparate in vivo impact of the chemosensitizer dipyridamole on the therapeutic index of cisplatin, carboplatin, and etoposide. Proc Am Assoc Cancer Res 32:374, 1991.
86. Sakaguchi Y, Emi Y, Maehara Y, Kohnoe S, and Sugimachi K. Combined treatment of adriamycin and dipyridamole inhibits lung metastasis of B16 melanoma cells in mice. Eur Surg Res 22:213–218, 1990.
87. Cao SS, and Zhen YS. Potentiation of antimetabolite antitumor activity in vivo by dipyridamole and amphotericin B. Cancer Chemother Pharmacol 24:181–186, 1989.
88. Isonishi S, Kirmani S, Kim S, Plaxe S, Braly PS, McClay EF, and Howell SB. Phase I and pharmacokinetic trial of intraperitoneal etoposide in combination with the multidrug-resistance-moulding agent dipyridamole. J Natl Cancer Inst 83:621–626, 1991.
89. Goel R, Sanga R, and Howell SB. Pharmacologic basis for the use of dipyridamole to increase the selectivity of intraperitoneally delivered methotrexate. Cancer Chemother Pharmacol 25:167–172, 1989.
90. Shalinsky DR, Andreef M, and Howell SB. Modulation of drug sensitivity by dipyridamole in multidrug resistant tumor cells in vitro. Cancer Res 50:7537–7543, 1990.
91. Shalinsky DR, and Howell SB. Modulation of vinblastine sensitivity by dipyridamole in multidrug resistant fibrosarcoma cells lacking mdrl expression. Proc Am Assoc Cancer Res 32:374, 1991.

Index